# Implementing primary health care

# IMPLEMENTING PRIMARY HEALTH CARE

## Experiences since Alma-Ata

Pieter Streefland and Jarl Chabot (eds.)

Royal Tropical Institute

Royal Tropical Institute
Rural Development Programme
Primary Health Care Section
Mauritskade 63
1092 AD Amsterdam
020-5688711

CIP-GEGEVENS KONINKLIJKE BIBLIOTHEEK, DEN HAAG

Implementing

Implementing primary health care : experiences since
Alma-Ata / P. Streefland and J. Chabot (eds.). -
Amsterdam : Royal Tropical Institute. - Ill.
ISBN 90-6832-034-3
SISO 601.5 UDC 614(1-77) NUGI 742
Trefw.: gezondheidszorg : Derde Wereld.


Cover design: Ad van Helmond
Printer: ICG Printing, Dordrecht

# Table of contents

# Preface

I am told that Einstein has said that 'the true sense of science is to reconcile the irreconcilable'.

The true sense of Primary Health Care also implies reconciling irreconcilables such as:
- to reconcile the moral imperative of *health equity* through a coherent application of health promotion, disease prevention, cure and rehabilitation with the irreconcilable inequity inherent in the operational dynamics of isolated curative medicine;
- to reconcile the supply of *appropriate technology* with the irreconcilable professional and popular demand for inappropriate technology;
- to reconcile the huge health benefits originating from *intersectoral synergies* with the irreconcilable vested interests in confusing health with medicine;
- to reconcile the demystifying force of *community participation* with the irreconcilable mystifying medical power.

Paraphrasing Einstein: the true sense of the continuous health struggle towards 2000 and beyond lies in our capacity to move towards the above reconciliations through a process of consensus aiming at the highest level of truth for the sake of the common good. This book - *Implementing Primary Health Care* - contributes very significant building blocks to this consensus process. It thereby also contributes towards preventing today's primary health care dogmas from becoming tomorrow's primary health care doubts.

Our health struggle is, in my opinion, beautifully expressed by Piet Hein in his Grook, inspired by Einstein:

'*We who are fighting to realize dreams*
*ask for the task of uniting extremes*'.

H. Mahler

Secretary General, International Planned Parenthood Federation
Director General Emeritus, World Health Organization

# Introduction

'Health for All by the year 2000' was the aim of the primary health care (PHC) strategy formulated by the Alma-Ata Conference in 1978. This conference, organised by the World Health Organization and UNICEF and attended by their member nations, was an outgrowth of changes in the perception of health: a shift from the earlier view of health as the result of combatting disease by biomedical means, to a new emphasis on the social and economic context of health.

The Alma-Ata strategy (see Appendix I) focused attention on PHC - the concept of 'essential health care made accessible at a cost that the country and community can afford'. Five basic principles were set out: equity, participation, appropriate technology, prevention, and an intersectoral approach to public health problems. The Alma-Ata Conference has greatly influenced national policies on improving and expanding health services. Countries that adopted the PHC strategy have begun translating the strategy into workable programmes, including a broad spectrum of activities: mother and child health, including nutrition and family spacing; provision of essential drugs; drinking water and sanitation; immunisation; health promotion and elementary curative care. Formulation and implementation of these 'primary health care' programmes has been supported by donor countries and multilateral agencies, which have provided money, ideas, and technical assistance.

As implementation began, a number of important issues surfaced. These have affected the shaping of PHC in the field and have also been the subject of much scholarly and managerial discussion. One such issue is the interface between BHS (basic health services) and CBHC (community based health care). In many developing countries the implementation of PHC began with the introduction and strengthening of CBHC via recruitment and training of village health workers and village health committees. Strengthening the BHS and building up the interrelationship with the CBHC - areas that are critical to the long-term support of CBHC - have received far less emphasis and often, in fact, have lagged behind.

Another issue concerns the form and contents of PHC itself. This is a strategic issue: what is the most effective means of achieving 'health for all'? New medical technologies in areas such as immunisation and control of diarrhoeal diseases, in combination with an emphasis on cost-effectiveness of interventions, have formed the basis for views and approaches that together have been called 'selective' PHC. This approach includes large scale intervention programmes, such as the expanded programme on immunisation, which are advocated on the basis of their considerable effectiveness in terms of the number of infant or child deaths prevented and the rapidity with which the programmes have an effect. Opponents of such 'selectiveness', however, point to possible neglect of long-term public health improvement, because funds and personnel are diverted from the regular health services. In the long run, they argue, sustained improvement in public health will be best achieved by a comprehensive strategy, even if this implies a slower process of implementation.

The international context of national PHC programmes is a third issue. This refers to the extent and way the (financial) policy of donors has influenced the implementation of PHC programmes within countries. Undeniably the influence of donors on the shaping of national PHC policies has been considerable; they often call the tune by first formulating and next applying their own criteria when providing support. Hence national governments have been stimulated to simply adapt their policies to such criteria, instead of formulating their own proposals and using these as a basis for negotiations with donors.

Such major issues, plus the practical problems that crop up in the process of implementing PHC at the district level and below, were the subject of discussions during a workshop held in Amsterdam in December 1988 on the occasion of the tenth anniversary of the Alma-Ata conference. The workshop was hosted by the PHC group of the Royal Tropical Institute, and was attended by about 80 technical advisors, health care staff from the field involved in implementing PHC, and representatives from donor agencies and national governments. Major inputs for the group discussions were statements for debate submitted by technical advisors, and papers on specific PHC projects, written by people involved in their implementation.

After the successful workshop, the PHC group decided to prepare English and French editions of a publication, including:

- the brief state-of-the-art papers prepared by the technical advisors who contributed to the workshop; and
- a number of case studies of PHC projects, based on workshop papers.

This publication is meant for health care staff involved in implementing PHC, including nurses, midwives, doctors, teaching staff, social scientists and others.

Both editions open with five contributions on four major themes in PHC (the case studies included in the French and English versions, however, differ). In Chapter one Susan Rifkin and Gill Walt discuss the *political context of PHC*. Their contribution focuses on the five basic principles of PHC formulated at Alma-Ata. For each principle, the authors consider the achievements of past years and the challenges that lie ahead. They conclude by mentioning some of the hard lessons of the past, which include that PHC is an ever evolving process, and that the importance of the social and cultural environment make it impossible to use replicable models or blueprints in PHC.

The second and third chapters focus on the *interrelation between the BHS and CBHC*. In Chapter two, Harry van Balen looks at this issue from the angle of the BHS, using examples from his broad experience in Francophone Africa. He discusses the importance of bringing about interactions between the rationality of the people and the rationality of the health workers. He shows that such interaction can be successful only if the following elements are taken into consideration: the demands of the people, the social cost of the underlying problem, the effectiveness of the people's solution, the effectiveness of the solution the BHS can offer, and the effort required to make both available solutions work. In Chapter three Pieter Streefland and Jarl Chabot take the CBHC as a point of departure in looking at the interface between this level of PHC and the BHS. They first provide a definition of CBHC, pointing out that the concept may be used in a broad sense, which includes a broad spectrum of health care activities at village level, and in a more narrow sense, specifically including activities of village health workers (VHWs) and village health committees. Subsequently their contribution systematically discusses the dynamics and lessons of CBHC in the narrower sense, touching upon e.g. the composition of village health committees, payment of VHWs, enhancement of the continuity of CBHC and improvement of its relationship with the BHS.

Chapter four, written by Fred Abbatt, concentrates on *personnel development and training*. Looking at past achievements and identifying areas that must be strengthened in the time to come, Abbatt discusses such topics as the implications of the tremendous increase in the number of health workers, consequences of changes in teaching methods and teaching materials, and the importance of in-service training. Among priorities for the future he includes increasing the competence of trainers of health workers and raising the status of health manpower training.

In Chapter five, which concludes the first part of the book, Lucy Gilson addresses the important issue of *financing systems in PHC*. This non-technical exploration of financing issues covers factors that are and have been an influence on the economic basis of PHC policy implementation in developing countries, the way in which existing resources to support PHC are actually used, and alternative possibilities for financing systems that can sustain the implementation of PHC in the years to come.

The seven case studies of PHC projects that follow have been written by authors reporting on their own experiences with project implementation. The seven chapters cover three continents: three projects are situated in Anglophone Africa, three in Asia and one in Latin America. Though the projects have in common that all have been initiated on the basis of the PHC strategy, they differ in emphasis and because of adaptation to specific social and cultural conditions. Each is included because we think it may contribute to an understanding of the process of implementing PHC, and may help readers to improve their work in PHC. The emphasis on the *process* of implementation implies that we have chosen to present the case studies without much quantitative information on mortality, morbidity, or performance of the health care staff.

A PHC project in the Northern part of Somalia is described in Chapter six by Chris Bentley. He outlines and analyses the implications of implementing PHC in a peripheral area without an existing basic health services structure. Moreover, the target group of the project where he worked as an advisor included both nomadic and settled peoples, which implied that the project structure and activities required careful tailoring to specific problems and possibilities. In Chapter seven, Eli Nangawe discusses a project among the Maasai in Tanzania that faced rather similar problems. His paper highlights how the project contributed to positive change in the situation of Maasai women, and provides us with valuable insight regarding the process of community participation. Chapter eight, by Jan Willem Harnmeijer, focuses on the issue of recurrent costs in PHC projects and programmes. On the basis of his experience in implementing PHC in the Western Province of Zambia, Harnmeijer discusses the financing of recurrent costs, paying ample attention to important factors like equity, as well as ability and willingness to pay.

The three contributions from Asia begin with a paper by Mustaque Chowdhury (Chapter nine) on the experience of one of the really large indigenous non-governmental development organisations in the developing world. BRAC in Bangladesh is implementing PHC via a staff of more than 3,000 women and men, and covers thousands of villages. Chowdhury discusses how BRAC began with a comprehensive form of PHC, but had to abandon this because it was not possible to realise equitable care in the villages, due to large differences in power and income. The organisation next got involved in large scale selective programmes, especially in promoting oral rehydration therapy. BRAC is still pursuing this approach, but at present is once again trying to further a more comprehensive form of PHC.

In Chapter ten, Sr. Sara Kaithathara gives a very personal account of her experience in working with village health workers in Orissa State, Eastern India. She describes a methodology that uses the skills, knowledge and efforts of the villagers themselves to improve their health conditions. She points out that this requires the health staff to have not only a basic attitude of confidence in people and their possibilities, but also an ability to look critically at their own outlook and prejudices. Chapter eleven also takes experience with community based health care as a point of departure. Magdalena Barcelon and Anita Hardon give a clear presentation of the way PHC principles have been realised in Community Based Health Programs in the Philippines. Though many aspects of these comprehensive programs are discussed, community participation and the role of community health workers receive special attention. It is also made clear that the conditions that prevail in many parts of the country due to militarisation put a great strain on the programs. In this respect there are parallels with the situation in Somalia, where civil war has wiped out much of the achievements described by Chris Bentley in the sixth chapter.

Finally, in Chapter twelve Patricia Dueñas describes experience with training health promoters in Colombia, with special attention to the training of health volunteers from the Indian minority in the province of Chocó. The process of training health promoters before Alma-Ata is contrasted with that after 1978, with a focus on the conceptual difference between education and training.

## Chapter 1

# The political context of primary health care

*Gill Walt and Susan Rifkin*

The 1978 Alma-Ata declaration crystalised many post-war experiences in health care, particularly in the developing countries. From the political chaos of post-war Europe emerged a period of global retrenchment in which conflicts of ideologies and conflicts over political control sharpened. The establishment of Communist China and the struggle for independence of the colonial world not only marked a new political reality but brought into focus universal values of liberation and concern for the oppressed. The calls for social justice and equity permeated all spheres of political and social life in both developing and developed countries.

In the field of health, this situation gave rise to the concept of health development. When Gunnar Myrdal wrote about 'investment in man', he removed the idea of health expenditure as a bottomless pit of disease treatment and pointed to its value in the development of people for increased production. One result was that the constitution of the WHO (World Health Organisation), which states that 'health is not merely the absence of disease' took on a new meaning. It became more acceptable to suggest that health was both a consequence of and a contribution to political and social order, and that health was not solely the result of the availability of medical services.

The concept of health development has many facets. Initially, in the 1950s, concern focused on the establishment of health care systems in newly emerging independent countries: the former colonial powers had established hospitals mainly for their armies and expatriates in urban settings, but the majority of people lived in scattered rural villages without access to curative institutions. By the 1960s, a new dimension was added when the UN called for a 'new economic order'. This moved the development focus from increased industrial production to concern with people's basic needs, including shelter, food, clothing, safe water, education and health care. In health care, a breed of doctors arrived who looked up from their surgical tables and consulting desks and saw that the future of good health lay not in individual treatment but in community development.

It was the experience of the 1960s, with its profound idealism, its questioning of traditional values, and its courage to challenge old orders that laid the basis for the new strategies for health development of the 1970s. Within this decade prominent people with professional prestige and ability to communicate came to the fore with ideas about the future of health care. Many of these ideas were investigated and taken up by the

World Health Organisation, the technical and professional body of the United Nations concerned with medical and health matters. By 1972, the WHO had brought to its executive board ideas about revamping health services to focus on the problems of those most in need. By 1978, primary health care was formalised and accepted by the World Health Assembly as the future of health care, embodying a conceptual recognition of good health as a result of socioeconomic factors and social justice. This was a dramatic contrast to the pre-war period, when medical professionals sought scientific solutions to disease problems as the means for health improvement.

## PHC today: achievements and challenges

In combination, the five principles of PHC - equity, prevention, appropriate technology, intersectoral action and community participation - represent a philosophy of health in which health improvements for the majority of the world's population depend more on political will than on technological improvements. PHC also depends upon the luxury of time and financial resources to pursue the strategy. While both were available in the 1960s, the oil crises of the mid-1970s so altered the world economy that, by the mid-1980s, available money to buy time for experimentation was in very short supply. It might be seen as ironic that as a new health paradigm emerged the resources needed to test it rapidly disappeared.

Ten years after Alma-Ata and ten years before the end of the century, how has PHC fared? What are its successes and what are its challenges? And what will determine whether these challenges are met? In the following pages, PHC will be reviewed and answers to the first and second questions will be attempted in the context of each of the PHC principles. The final part of this paper will address the questions of what determines whether these challenges are met and what lessons we have learned from the past.

*Equity*

It might well be argued that in the Alma-Ata declaration, equity was accepted as the main principle of PHC. The new predominance of the concerns of accessibility, acceptability and affordability of health services reflected the importance of the ideal of social justice in health. Experience showed that health improvements for nations and societies depended on ensuring that health resources reached those traditionally without access. In turn, this demanded ways to redistribute these resources. Inspiration for equity came from the Chinese experience, where the political will of the new Communist government put health care for all high on the social agenda, and radically altered disease patterns without enormous extra financial input. Inspiration was also gathered from small NGO programmes with charismatic leaders, committed personnel and clear visions of the future.

Ten years since Alma-Ata, equity still has high priority on the health agenda. It remains a consistent goal of national governments, of donor agencies, of the UN and of NGOs. However, the translation of the principle into practice has not been as simple as merely transferring resources. Both resources and political commitment have been lacking in a majority of situations. As a result, the development of PHC has relied on the four other principles as mechanisms to ensure equity. These principles have come to focus both on shifting resources and on creating structures to insure that these resources are utilised. For the future, the preservation of PHC demands the continual pursuit of equity, and this challenge demands securing the mechanisms by which this goal can be realised.

*Prevention*

The principle of prevention became important to PHC because of both cost and human concern. The argument that it was more cost effective to prevent disease than to continue to treat the same person for that disease over again was persuasive. In addition, the idea of 'investment in man' demanded that people stay healthy to participate in production.

The emphasis on prevention has made an important contribution to the principle of equity in the less developed countries. It has demanded and gained a concern for a shift of expenditure from urban teaching hospitals to rural health centres, where prevention claims significant amounts of time from both providers and beneficiaries. In many countries, it has contributed to a restructuring of the Ministry of Health, where preventive and curative activities have been integrated. It also has ensured that resources are targeted to the prevention of diseases (to which the poor are most vulnerable) through promotion of mass awareness and immunisation campaigns.

Prevention has enabled progress toward PHC by contributing to activities that help those most vulnerable to illness to avoid its consequences. It has emphasised and gained resources for health education and, in this context, for concerns about changing health behaviours rather than merely providing information. It has increased the awareness of the medical professional of the benefits of promoting prevention, with the result that real attempts have been made to review educational curricula and to increase cooperation among health and medical staff.

The greatest challenge to prevention as a mechanism to insure equity is the increasing demand for expensive, individual curative care. This demand is not only a result of rising expectations of the population for access to modern health technologies, but also of the fact that health is rarely perceived as a priority unless someone is ill. It is complicated by the realisation of two impending crises that have emerged in the last 10 years. First, rapid urban growth, with its impoverished populations who lack political, social and/or economic access to the benefits of prevention, increases the pressure of demands for curative treatment rather than community care. Second, the emergence of AIDS as the major epidemic of the latter half of the 20th century is diverting scarce health resources to care for large numbers of terminally ill people. For the future, prevention is a critical mechanism for ensuring equity: through allocations to community health concerns, it secures funds for and focuses on those who lack access to increasingly costly medical treatment.

*Appropriate technology*
In the PHC context, emphasis on appropriate technology has highlighted the need to release health allocations from the straightjacket of buying increasingly advanced and increasingly expensive medical 'high tech'. By arguing for the accumulation and application of simple solutions to practical problems that plague the majority of the world's population, this shifted some support for medical expenditures away from highly sophisticated curative institutions and training of specialised staff, to the provision of more funds to care for prevention and cure of the most prevalent diseases.

Achievements in this area include the successful search for - and acceptance of - simple and appropriate solutions to large health problems. Examples include the relatively widespread use of oral rehydration therapy for diarrhoeal disease (see Chowdhury on Bangladesh, Chapter 9), the use of simple weighing scales and arm circumference measurements to help identify poorly nourished children and to assist mothers in recognising the problem, and, in some countries, the construction of comparatively cheap ventilated pit latrines. These technologies have reduced costs of individual interventions as well as giving educational benefits, helping to change health behaviours. They have helped the poor gain some improvements in an area where professional concerns and demands for technological advancement often support developments that address the problems of the relatively few.

In the area of appropriate technology, the challenge will continue to be gaining scarce resources for the health problems of the poor majority in the face of pressure from the medical profession and the industrial technologists to advance the frontiers of medicine. This challenge will be complicated by changing disease patterns, since treating hypertension, heart disease, cancers and AIDS (as we have noted) can demand sophisticated technology. It will entail a struggle to assure people that PHC and appropriate technology are not medicine for the poor but a legitimate and critical approach to massive health improvements. It will require a fight to preserve the present gains and to continue the mandate to search for innovations. For the future, appropriate technology is critical not only because it makes a practical contribution but also because it ensures the ability of lay people to keep health technologies in their own hands and to maintain independence from the professional.

*Intersectoral action*
After the definition of the causes of poor health expanded to include the socioeconomic environment, it became critical to identify the precise nature of this environment and the sectors that had resources to help improve the situation.
The health sector could set up new health service units, but problems of poor nutrition also needed to be addressed by the agricultural sector, problems of water and sanitation by water resources, and problems of health education by departments of education and community development. Proponents of PHC argued that the problems of the poor could only be solved by bringing resources together, not by dividing the problems and allocating them to separate government departments. The sum of total resources was seen to be greater than the addition of individual parts.

Perhaps the greatest achievement in developing this mechanism for equity has been the creation of awareness among the different sectors of their influence on health care and health improvements. Discussions among various ministries have taken place at national levels in some countries and problems have been identified. In the area of intersectoral action, activities and joint planning can be found in cities, where, at the municipal level, problems and their interrelationships are more obvious. In rural areas, different departments often work closely together by necessity and due to personal relationships. The NGOs provide experiences on a small scale of instances where rural development programmes have been jointly planned and executed among different sectors.

The challenge in intersectoral action is still to define areas of common concern and action. While this item is high on the health agenda, many other sectors assign health a low priority within the national agenda; as a result, urging such action is often seen as an attempt of the health ministry to dictate actions and commandeer resources for its own control. This view is sustained by the fact that health is still often seen as the purview of medical doctors, whose concerns are identified as disease, not development. In the future, attempts at intersectoral action will face a technologically focused world with fewer resources and more competition among sectors for control. Given a lack of solid examples of cases where an intersectoral approach has worked on a large scale, plus the existing weak infrastructure in many countries, it will be increasingly difficult to argue for support and credibility. The contribution of intersectoral action to ensuring equity may well be minimal.

*Community participation*

Community participation has been called the key to PHC, because it has been seen as the mechanism that ensured that health care beneficiaries became involved in the decision making process of health care priorities and resource allocations. (See for example the contributions of Barcelon, Kaithathara, and Nangawe.) Participation not only challenged the medical professionals' role, but also attempted to empower people to take political and individual control over their own lives. Its advocacy particularly focused on the poor and oppressed, using health as an entry point for gaining social justice.

Community participation emerged as the principle with the highest profile. Not only is it the most controversial, promoting a role for the layman in health care, but also it is a focus of action for wider community development and, in some cases, political activities. Achievements have included effective advocacy for the role of the individual, especially the impoverished, in health choices; the creation of new structures, including community health committees and community health workers, to insure these rights; and the establishment of the principle as a key factor in a range of health improvement interventions from mass campaigns to communicable disease control. As a necessary factor for future public health planning in all countries, its importance is becoming increasingly acknowledged.

Community participation is a complicated concept for which no standard definition can be agreed. It is often used to describe activities in which community people merely benefit, but make no contribution to the decision making process. This situation is most apparent in many national community health worker schemes where, instead of developing into methods for community input for resource decisions, the schemes have been co-opted by health ministries as a means to extend health services to peripheral communities. Other health programmes have used community participation as a means to conduct mass immunisation campaigns, to gain contributions of resources to programmes, and/or to promote better service utilisation. In these activities decisions are taken by the professionals, and the community participates by accepting these decisions. In the context of PHC, the future challenge is to build or strengthen existing structures to break the monopoly on decision making by medical professionals and insure a process where laymen gain experience and confidence to actively participate in their own and their community's health improvements.

## Meeting the challenges

Will these challenges be met? The answer lies in policy decisions in three separate arenas.

First is the international arena. Here the policy makers include national governments and bilateral and international donors. The financial crisis has forced many national governments to choose policies of financial restructuring, which has compromised both social policies and the commitment to equity. One result is that the international climate at present is not conducive to cooperation or promotion of policies of equity. Cost recovery and privatisation of national health services command attention. Emphasis on the impact of health technologies rather than processes for change are gaining increasing importance. Another result is that countries now rely even more on donor support for additional monetary resources and for means to maintain and expand the mechanisms and structures to ensure development for the poor. If this support is not forthcoming, and if monetary constraints limit the time and space necessary for a reorientation of governments concerning approaches to health improvements, PHC will loose valuable ground.

In the second, the national arena, policy depends on national governments alone. While resource allocation to the health and social sectors is critical, this alone is not sufficient to meet the challenges of preserving PHC. The main determinant of successful PHC development will depend on the existence of a strong and capable health systems infrastructure, which includes development of good management structures and skills and strong methods of monitoring and evaluating. The infrastructure will also have to include mechanisms for decentralisation, in order to realise both rational resource allocation and the potential for mobilisation of political commitment. Local governments will need to have both money and control to meet local problems, which otherwise will be overrun by national political considerations and priorities. If strong infrastructures are not developed and if decentralisation cannot be realised, PHC will flounder.

In the third, the local arena, meeting the challenges depends on maintaining and creating structures to insure local participation. These structures cannot be merely an additional layer of health workers to extend services, but should include structures for decision making that insure the participation process and the dialogue between professionals and laymen. These structures will need to be responsive to special groups within the community. Women's needs must be reflected, and those of people at the very periphery of community life, the old, the disabled and the very poor. If these structures are not established, decisions at other levels about preserving equity will not take root. If at the local level a strong base, which ensures participation of all members and channels for dialogue and action at the national and international level, is not developed and maintained, PHC will be seriously endangered.

*Lessons from the past*

Meeting the challenges of PHC for the future will depend on studying and learning from the past. The decades leading up to Alma-Ata and the ten years following provide a rich tapestry of experience from which valuable insights have emerged. The 'Alma-Ata Ten Years After' workshop hosted by the Royal Tropical Institute, on which this book is based, put forward some of the most important lessons. Among them are the following:

*PHC is contextual.* PHC has not provided a single, replicable model of health care which, like a campaign for smallpox eradication or measles immunisation, can be repeated in different communities and different countries. PHC has emerged from local experiences. As the definition in the Alma-Ata declaration suggests, PHC depends on making health care acceptable, affordable and available to all members of the community. How this goal translates depends on existing social, economic and political conditions in each locality. Readjustment rather than replication of programmes is a key feature of successful PHC.

*PHC is a process.* PHC is a comprehensive approach to health improvement. It is not merely a selective health intervention aimed at improving health status for a target group. Being a process, it develops over time and changes to meet new situations. As a process, it needs financial resources available for a long term strategy. The struggle for monetary contributions between those who want immediate results and those who see the value of a long term commitment has plagued both the definition and the programme support of PHC. Given the atmosphere of economic austerity, the struggle is by no means concluded. As a result, there are continued demands to translate the process into a product, and to pressure advocates of PHC to clearly describe the processes they support.

*PHC is based on high service quality and commitment.* PHC is still seen as basically a delivery of a health service. Even though many countries have expanded their primary level services into remote rural areas and provided health workers to neglected groups, the credibility of this service still depends on the quality of care and the concern of the health providers. Where services are weak and staff uninterested, PHC has been discredited as second class care. Where services have been delivered well, confidence in the health staff has enabled these people to become involved in and often lead wider community development projects. Quality and commitment demand a reorientation in the goals and education of health personnel. (In this regard, see also Kaithathara and Nangawe.)

*PHC is built on dialogue and information.* PHC succeeds where lay people and health professionals are able to establish confidence and respect for each other in order to solve health problems with complex causes. This process of dialogue ensures local concerns are heard and a forum is available to negotiate solutions. The dialogue is greatly enhanced when both groups have information on which to base their views and opinions. Health information networks are critical to enable PHC to function well. Where these networks have been formalised, information has been more systematically available and more easily accessible. In this process, both dialogue and dissemination of information strengthen the basis of PHC and the infrastructures critical to its development.

PHC, in important part, must be preserved and promoted not only through the dissemination of experiences, but also through the analysis of concepts and methodologies. There is a need to provide an understanding of experiences, and research and publications are necessary to meet this need. Research must to be scientific but also participatory and action oriented. Research undertaken jointly by academic institutions and field programme staff, followed by proper dissemination of information, is one positive way to meet this need.

## Chapter 2

# An adequate interface with the community: the contribution of the basic health services

*Harry van Balen*

In the decades preceding Alma-Ata, health care providers, health service organisers, governments and non-governmental organisations alike faced problems as they tried to make adequate health care available to all. They found solutions as well as disappointments.

During the fifties, hospitals were built and equipped and doctors (preferably specialists) were trained in order to make the successful new medical technology available to more and more people. Technical progress aroused enormous expectations: worldwide problems such as malaria were to be eradicated, provided the required resources were made available.

The declaration of human rights, the restoration of democracies, and the concern for social justice resulted in systems of social security in many countries: national taxes or (compulsory) insurance schemes were to guarantee free access to health services when needed. In the late fifties and sixties, there was growing awareness of the importance of the operational aspects of health care. The decentralisation of health services, with simple technology implemented by less qualified health personnel, was introduced. All too often this decentralisation was organised as an extension of the centralised services, a second-best solution for people living too far away from the central towns, to be used as long as 'really good' service was not accessible.

With health care a human right, even in poor countries, governments developed free health care systems, responding to professionally determined health needs. Yet people did not react as health workers thought they should. Health education came into fashion. This was, to a great extent, a form of social marketing, a one way communication, trying to convince people to do what health workers considered was good for them. Meanwhile other structures met the demand for care: drug hawkers, drugstore keepers, and all sorts of clever healers.

In the seventies, it became obvious in many rich countries that a social security system that encourages over-consumption of medical technology alienates people from their human condition. Social security succeeded so well that it jeopardised the autonomy of the individual, the family and the people in health matters. Some groups, eager to safeguard their capacity for autonomous choice in health matters, demanded general practitioners and health services capable of establishing human relations, to interact with patients and their families.

In poor countries it became obvious that free care cannot be delivered in an acceptable way when resources are insufficient. Many local initiatives, often by non-governmental organisations, showed that reasonable patient charges improve the acceptability of health care, simply by making essential drugs and other material available. Likewise, it was shown that real dialogue, real interaction between the health care providers and the people increases autonomy and self-help (Newell, 1975).

## Alma-Ata

The Alma-Ata declaration in 1978 was the culmination of a long period of field work and research concerning the optimisation of health care, sustained by a long-term vision. The definition of primary health care (article 6 of the Alma-Ata declaration; see Appendix I) evokes a dynamic equilibrium between people's autonomy and responsibility on the one hand, and the effectiveness and efficiency of the health services, on the other. It makes a plea for participatory decision making in health matters. Such continuous participation requires an 'interface', channels of dynamic interaction between health care providers and the people.

The rationale of the health services is based on an analysis of the suffering caused by health problems and the possibility of reducing or suppressing this suffering via health care or health promotion. On the other hand, people's readiness to influence their health is embedded in a complete value system. Improving health is not always a priority. People will not accept efforts required to improve health that jeopardise the realisation of values they consider to be more important.

The function of the 'interface' is to bring about interaction between the rationale of the people and the rationale of the health workers in such a way that all elements are taken into account in looking for solutions: the demand of the people, the social cost of the underlying problem and the effectiveness of the people's solutions, as well as the effectiveness of the health services' solutions and the respective efforts required.

## Miscalculations in implementing interfaces after Alma-Ata

*Too rapid scaling-up of local successes.* There is no doubt that a dynamic interaction between the two rationales often takes place, albeit mostly on a small scale. When applied on a large scale, the complexity of the system or the pace of behavioral change have too often been overlooked. Indeed, some governments or funding agencies committed to primary health care have looked for rapid solutions, for 'instant success'. Local projects have expanded too rapidly into national systems. This has happened for political rather than for pragmatic reasons (Berman et al., 1987). As a consequence, neither system adjustment nor adaptation to local situations was possible. Such programmes defined at national (or even international) level were pushed through at local level, often including a fake interface. In many countries, primary health care even became a vertical programme with its own structure, alongside the apparently undisturbed 'modern' health services and the existing traditional health system (Senghor, 1984).

In Niger a successful interaction between the health services and local communities was observed in the sixties (Belloncle and Fournier, 1975; Newell, 1975). At grass roots level, villagers themselves decided to increase their own capacity to tackle problems, beginning from a list of problems covering all sectors of development. In those villages where a health problem was selected, the health services were consulted to find out how the village's capacity for tackling those problems could be improved. As a result of the interaction, a type of community based health care developed: a village pharmacy, one or two village health workers, one or two treasurers and sometimes a health committee. After a few years, experience showed that the continuation of those initiatives required an intensive interaction between first line health services and the villages, which could be done only in a very limited number of villages.

At the end of the seventies it was decided to expand those local successes into a national system (Van Balen, 1987). Unfortunately, programme developers acted like people who, admiring a nice butterfly and wanting to get many more of them without delay, open up the pupae to speed up the development of the butterflies. Villages were to imitate the model. In order to reach the target (number of villages to be served) small financial incentives were offered to the village health worker. The decision to increase community capacity to tackle a problem selected by themselves was no longer a real grassroots level decision with the participation of all. Village health workers were no longer facilitators of a village initiative, nor a channel for village communication with the health services. Instead, they became executors of a top-down programme, outposts of the health services. Although they were not really familiar with the rationale of the health services, they were expected to express this rationale in their interaction with the villagers. The supportive capacity of the peripheral health services had not been considered, and it very quickly became incapable of keeping up a dynamic interaction with all the people involved. False expectations, many drop outs, and deviation to mere selling of drugs on demand were the results.

Attempts to scale up a successful project have been recorded all over the world. The urge to realise 'equity', to make health care and health education universally accessible, has superceded considerations such as efficacy, sustainability, people's values and demands, and the capacity of the health services to respond to expectations. With respect to communication and participatory decision making, it has often been counterproductive.

*Overlooking know-how.* A personal observation in Benin (Mercenier, 1986) illustrates how imposing a centrally conceived standard model for involving villagers can conflict with the bottom-up development of know-how in health matters.

A few weeks before our visit to a village of about 500 inhabitants, villagers had been asked to select two people to be trained as village health workers. The main objectives of the training programme were the development of capacity to treat fever cases with chloroquine, to disinfect wounds, to use oral rehydration, to apply eye ointment and to administer simple analgesics.

The conversation we had with a group of about 20 inhabitants of the village was very informal. It revealed that all knew the doses of chloroquine for children of different ages. Moreover, the drug was being sold in that same village by a hawker at a price comparable to what the future village health workers would ask. Questioned on the way to deal with wounds, the villagers referred to a male adult. He knew the leaves to apply to wounds. He agreed that this sort of dressing was not very effective in the event of deep wounds. For these cases he had developed a new technique. He crushes the leaves, mixes them with powder from red capsules (tetracycline) sold by the hawker, and applies this to the wound. He has noted much better results since using this technique.

The next topic was diarrhoea. For this problem the villagers referred to another male adult. His treatment is a stiff decoction of goyava leaves. In his opinion, liquid intake should be limited as much as possible, because 'liquid keeps diarrhoea going'. A conversation with the medical staff about what a dehydrated child looks like led him to agree that it resembles an empty drinking bag. The idea of adding more water to the decoction administered to such a child in order to prevent its complete flattening was found to deserve serious consideration. Even if the 'diarrhoea expert' was not completely convinced, at least an open discussion began, which he might remember next time he is confronted with such a case.

Toward the end of the meeting it struck us that two youngsters had been listening all the time without participating in the conversation. When we asked who they were, it seemed they were the two persons to be trained as village health workers.

Two obvious lessons can be taken from these observations. Firstly, regular communications between competent first line health workers and villagers (for instance after a mother and child health session), grafting new knowledge and insights onto existing capacities, can increase the self-reliance of the community and their understanding of the complementarity of the health services.

Secondly, training village health workers to adhere to a centrally standardised schedule overlooks the existing 'health culture'. It devotes the resources of the health services to the development of new structures that pay no attention to the recognised 'health care experts' of the village. This is not an appropriate approach, nor is it likely to bring about an integration between the rationale of the health services and that of the people.

*Reducing health committees to treasurers.* Health committees are another structure through which certain types of interaction between the community and the health services can take place. Committees may play a significant role in adjusting the health services to the felt needs of the people, and may facilitate participation in health services activities, including complementary financing. In this structure, unfortunately, interaction has often too exclusively focused on self financing for the health services. If cost recovery is the only concern of the committee, health services hesitate to reduce financial barriers for the poor. People are then discouraged from attempting self help, and health personnel are discouraged from devoting much time to communication with patients. If, moreover, the committee controlling the financial resources is composed of people whose primary concern is not the adequate functioning of the health services, then the people who use and pay for the service as well as health services staff may be betrayed; only a small fraction of the money collected by charging patients may be used to pay for services. When this happens, a potential communication channel is jeopardised.

*Overlooking people's demand for curative care.* At the beginning of the eighties a group of professionals put forward the idea of selective primary health care (Walsh and Warren, 1980). This idea is based on the illusion that the major health problems have a few causes that can be readily attacked, and that health care can be made acceptable without taking the demand of the people for curative care into account. In this approach one can only conceive of an interface between the people and the health services as an instrument for social marketing, for selling the services selected by the health professionals. There is no plan to use communication channels to slowly modify the functioning of health infrastructures, nor for a flexible strategy based upon the very real local health culture and the demand for care.

*Mere response to demand.* On the other hand, some initiatives were too exclusively based on the local health culture and demand: cooperatives, parishes, drug sellers and private practitioners, all organised health care which did not bother about irrationalities in the people's demand for care. They do not see the purpose of a continuous dialogue with the health services. Medical professionals are viewed as an external resource one calls upon for purely technical reasons (Rifkin and Walt, 1986; Walsh and Warren, 1980). Merely responding to concrete demands, without an ongoing exchange with the health services about the rationale of the demand, leads among other things to over-consumption, use of inefficient drugs, shopping around by anxious patients, discontinuity of care, etc.

*Hospitals as inappropriate urban interfaces.* Concern for equity had another logical consequence: it was thought that more efforts should be oriented toward the development of rural health care. Many countries can be proud of their networks of rural health centers and health posts, which have made health care and communication on health matters much more accessible to rural people. Unfortunately, however, urban hospitals - with their crowded outpatient departments and mother and child health clinics - were implicitly considered to be suitable health communications channels for urban dwellers. As a consequence, the development of urban first line health services, interacting with a limited and recognisable population, was neglected. This was a lost opportunity to create, in urban settings, an interface where the omnipotence of medical technology and of newly developed drugs could be demystified.

In summary, when planning a health service, capacity for communication with the target population should certainly be provided. But one should keep in mind that the interaction between the rationale of the health services and that of the population consists of a set of various and flexible communication channels at different levels. This interface cannot be reduced to village health workers, nor to health committees, nor to superficial contacts at the outpatient department nor to private practice. Nor can it be restricted to rural areas.

Moreover, participatory decisions must fit into an integrated system: while acting in accord with these decisions, health services must still be able to meet their commitments for direct service, as well as for supervision and logistic support.

## Structural problems of the health centre as interface

In spite of many faulty applications in the past, the PHC strategy remains of universal relevance. The realisation of comprehensiveness and accessibility will in the future continue to depend upon a participatory approach, even though the modes of application will vary with the cultural, social and economic context and will change in the course of time.

In order to implement the optimal mix of top-down and bottom-up planning, the World Health Organisation in 1987 formulated recommendations in Harare for 'Strengthening District Health Systems based on PHC'.

The rational organisation of an integrated health care system at district level indicates complementarity - not competition - between the professional rationale and the people's rationale of the system. If the system is to deliver comprehensive care, the first line health services are the privileged places where the interaction between these two rationales takes place. This first line must be complemented by second line services; they must not compete.

Establishing urban and rural networks of appropriate, accessible and acceptable first level health facilities brings the health services side of the interface as close as possible to the community, which must be seen as both beneficiary and participant. 'Appropriate' means here that in such a facility, the quality of the communication is as important as what is said; and that the empathy of the personnel is as important as technical skill.

*Minimum services necessary for a 'healthy' interface*

Given the importance of communication, the services organised at this level should first of all contribute to the development of a healthy relationship between the services and the people, based on mutual confidence. That is why it is important for services to give priority in their response to the needs felt by the community.

The demands of the people are best confronted at the clinic, but in order to contribute positively to interaction, staff must simultaneously adhere to professionally defined needs, which include the efficient use of drugs (so as to counterbalance misleading publicity), relieving anxiety, giving access to the referral level when required, and making a participatory decision (that is, taking the total human dimension of the patient into consideration).

Organising the care and active follow-up of chronic patients is a second priority. This involves much more than mere curative activity. The caseholding component is an excellent bridge to the more educational aspects of preventive care. Indeed, the caseholding of patients who no longer feel sick is an excellent opportunity for a health worker to sharpen and test capacity to communicate with people, because it concerns a small number of familiar individuals. It can be an indicator of capacity to communicate with the community at large with regard to more ambitious preventive and promotive goals. Caseholding provides an opportunity for self evaluation, by treating data which are relatively easily collected. It involves a systematic strategy of case retrieval, which includes home visits with specific objectives. The design of such a strategy implies the identification of a small, well-defined group of people, the environmental and cultural determinants of human behaviour, and means to exert positive influence.

Care and active follow-up of high risk groups also belongs in the minimum package for a first line health service. In any community, high risk groups can be identified. This might include people exposed to professional risks, e.g. agriculturists exposed to pesticides and industrial workers. Age groups, like old people or school children, might be included, or women who are pregnant or at risk from unwanted pregnancies.

Curative care, continuous care for chronic patients, including follow-up, and preventive care plus follow-up for high risk groups are the three basic services that respond to the existing felt needs of the community. First line health services responding to felt needs in these ways inspire the confidence required for building an interface with the community, and exemplify the health centre concept.

The technical level of the health centre should be sufficient to create confidence by responding satisfactorily to a significant part of felt priority needs. In other words, the technical level of a health centre should support the human relations aspects, which are a salient feature of care in first line health services. At the same time it should also satisfy the professional expectations of the health care workers.

Other functions, like environmental sanitation, community health education, housing, and systematic campaigns will develop gradually, as part of a long term process, but should result from the interaction between the health services and the community. They should not be planned before the real needs have been defined. This community diagnosis is a gradual and rather long term process. Health promotion activities should not be implemented before the community has recognised these needs and their relative priority.

*Structural conditions for establishing a health centre*

If the professionals in the district health system want to offer this holistic, continuous and integrated care as a part of first line health services, to promote a permanent dialogue between the people and the staff, and consequently to involve the people in the activities, a certain number of structural conditions must be established.

The first line health services structure, the health centre, should create maximum opportunities for access, in all respects (mental and cultural, as well as physical).

The optimal size and number of ‘health centers’ in a district will be a trade off between accessibility and technology. Easy access is a condition for good human relations. A certain level of technology is a condition for providing relevant care (complementing what people can do themselves).

*Population to be covered.* Clearly the size of the population covered will influence all other structural problems. There is a risk of focusing too much on geographical accessibility, which is the most easily measurable accessibility variable. Two extreme situations may arise.

Scattered population: here there is a risk that the health centre will be too small, with almost no relevant technology available. With small centres, physical accessibility will be good, but more frequent referrals to a unit that is more distant and therefore less accessible will be necessary. Moreover, supervision of too great a number of health centres by the supporting district staff may become inadequate. The alternative is a health centre that is slightly more distant but better equipped, and covers a larger population.

Dense population: here there is a risk that the health centre will be too big, with numerous staff, losing any capacity for holistic and continuous care. Such facilities are irrelevant. Not only do they jeopardise the human component of the health centre and decrease its quality of care, but also continuous direct access would flood it with simple problems that do not require that level of technology. Costs would be increased and in the long run even the technical quality of the hospital would be put in jeopardy.

In both situations the size of the population to be covered is a more relevant criterion than mere distance. If, in scarcely populated areas, this criterion would not ensure good geographical accessibility for the entire community, health centre workers may resort to extension of outreach facilities (subcentres, mobile services, village health workers).

This point underlines an advantage of the district approach, which leads to flexibility in interpreting national standards. These should be used as indicative averages, necessary for resource allocation.

*Size of the building.* The size of the building depends upon the interrelation between the size of the population, the size of the team and the level of technology. There are, however, a few general considerations:

• the design should be as simple as possible; it should respond to the needs of the services offered;

• it should particularly take into account the need for people to meet (e.g. health committees).

Meetings would preferably be held in an open place, and not behind closed doors. Here, however, one should take into account the availability of other community buildings (another advantage of district planning) as an opportunity to work with other sectors.

*Health centre team.* The best conditions for active interaction with the community are created if the health centre is staffed by a small integrated team, which means a team of health workers acting as a polyvalent whole. An integrated team is ideally composed of polyvalent health workers sharing, according to their qualification, a common responsibility for all health problems in the community. If the level of work requires specialised health workers, and if those workers are expected to work as a team, development of an intra-team communication system will be required. Eventually internal referrals will be needed to keep the team one integrated unit. However, the necessity for such a system creates additional human problems; it is more difficult to manage, and therefore increases the risk of failure.

Those who come to a health facility with multiple problems face a strong psychological barrier when each of the various workers they meet knows only one aspect of their problem. Being polyvalent is still the strength of the general practitioner working alone, and this experience should not be neglected.

Moreover, since health workers are professionals, their professional competence does differentiate them from the people; that in itself causes the gap PHC tries to bridge. It is therefore important to avoid unnecessary differences, e.g. cultural and social gaps, which would further prevent the development of the necessary empathetic relation. These gaps can be reduced by sharing the physical and social environment of the people, and thereby knowing the people in their environment. Finally, training in communication skills is as necessary as training in technical skills to give the staff the capacity needed to do their jobs.

*Financing.* Another structural problem to be solved in developing a sustainable interface between the health services and the people is financing. The self financing of the health centre by the target population in order to obtain the resources for a relevant level of functioning is also an excellent opportunity for participatory decision making. This aspect is developed in Chapter 5 of this reader. Regarding general structural problems of the health centre as an interface, see also Béthune, 1986; the Kasongo Project Team, 1980; Mercenier, 1986.

### Interaction between health services and the people

Once the necessary structural conditions have been realised, where should communication channels be established? The dialogue between health workers and the people should clearly not be a 'specialised' activity; further, it occurs at various levels.

*Talking with individuals.* At the individual level, the first but least often used opportunity is the clinic. Listening to the reactions of patients during diagnosis and prescription, making explanations and possibly adaptations to increase acceptability, is an excellent opportunity, because it takes place with a patient in a situation of felt need. It is limited, however, because the discussion may often not go beyond the patient's perceived problem, and may be biased by the patient's anxiety. But these defects decrease during the patient's second and third visits. It becomes very fruitful, for specific as well as for unspecific purposes, with chronic patients. Individual dialogue must also take place with users of preventive services, which enlarges the scope of dialogue to include many more health conditions than the curative situation.

*Chatting with small groups.* The next level of dialogue is in small groups. Here the interaction becomes a more organised activity. It might be at the health centre or in outreach clinics, with for example, animation sessions with users of preventive services, pregnant women attending the antenatal clinic, or mothers attending the well-baby clinic. The small groups might be families, when home visits are made for specific or non-specific purposes. For chronic patients, home visits which permit family sessions are very beneficial because, at that micro community level, this bridges the isolation of the individual chronic patient from his immediate social environment. For non-specific purposes, intra-home visits might easily be enlarged to include more than single families and become opportunities for dialogue with mini-communities at the neighbourhood or village level. Similarly, mother and child health clinics could be followed by dialogue with villagers interested or influential in health matters.

*Interacting with the community*. The previous dialogue situations, even those organised for small groups, aim at selected people. They do not create a dialogue with the community as a more or less organised whole. This systematic form of interaction is an absolute requirement for developing participatory decision making or community self management of a local health system. These levels of community participation require regular meetings with a 'health committee'. It doesn't matter whether the health committee is an autonomous body, whether it is an expression of a more general 'development committee' or whether the development committee acts as a health committee. What matters is that the health committee be as representative as possible of the community, which is not easy, because it involves a number of local socio-political considerations. Clearly, the level of self management that can be achieved depends on the level of representativeness of the health committee, and on the quality of community leadership it has been able to promote.

*Negotiation at the district level*. Finally, communication channels also have a role at district level, in the interaction between the people and the district health services.

Though dialogue with the community is a specific responsibility of the health centre, community issues are sometimes too complex to be tackled effectively by health centre workers. In such cases it may be necessary to involve higher level professional staff from the district level, to solve such complex issues at community level or to work with health committees. Intervention by district level staff is also relevant to problems concerning areas covered by more than one health centre.

However, when the support of this staff is required, their external contribution should not interfere with the relationship between the community and the local health workers. Therefore the health centre staff should not be bypassed. On the contrary, they should be continuously involved in the whole process, because it remains their responsibility.

On the other hand, community involvement at the health centre level (local communities) should be extended to the district level, where referrals are sent. Community involvement at the local level might be considered only a starting point, which must become the strong base for extension to the district. The dialogue at local level should prepare for this development, and be based on a clear view of the local community as only a part of a larger whole. The representativeness of the negotiating body at this level is more important than at the local level, because opportunities for direct communication are rare. The health staff at district level should be involved both directly and indirectly in the development and utilisation of the communication channels in the district.

## Conclusion

If they are developed simultaneously at the interface between the health services and the people, participation and rationalisation - the adjustment of the rationale of the people and the rationale of the health services - can bring equity and self-reliance into balance with effectiveness and efficiency, and contribute to a sustainable process that produces real improvements in the health of the people.

## References

Balen, H. van, 'Primaire Gezondheidszorg: geen bijkomend programma, maar een fundamentele aanpassing van het gezondheidssysteem'. *Mededelingen der Zittingen Koninklijke Academie voor Overzeese Wetenschappen*, vol. 33, no. 2 (1987) pp. 227-291.

Belloncle and Fournier, *Santé et développement en milieu rural africain*. Paris, Editions Ouvrières, 1975.

Berman, P.A., D.R. Gwatkin and S.E. Burger, 'Community-based health workers: head start or false start towards health for all?'. *Social Science and Medicine*, vol. 25 (1987), pp. 443-459.

Béthune, X. de, 'Primary Health Care and its alternative: selective activities on health status'. Working Paper 13, Antwerp, Institute Tropicale Médicine, 1986.

Kasongo Project Team, 'The Kasongo project'. *Annales de la Société Belge de Médecine Tropicale*, vol. 60, Supplément 1980.

Mercenier, P., 'The role of the health centre in the district health system based on primary health care'. Working document WHO, 1986.

Newell, K.W., 'Health by the people'. Geneva, World Health Organisation, 1975.

Rifkin, S. and G. Walt, 'Why health improves: defining the issues concerning comprehensive health care and selective primary health care'. *Social Science and Medicine*, vol. 23 (1986), pp. 559-566.

Senghor, D., 'Les soins de santé primaires. Révolution ou alibi?' *Famille et Développement*, vol. 28 (1984), pp. 34-58.

Walsh, J.A. and K.S. Warren, 'Selective Primary Health Care: an interim strategy for disease control in developing countries'. *Social Science and Medicine*, vol. 14C (1980) pp. 145-163.

Chapter 3

# Community based health care and the interface with the basic health services

*Pieter Streefland and Jarl Chabot*

Health care at the community level encompasses a broad range of activities and functions. To reach a better understanding of the inherent complexities, we may distinguish three categories of community level health care:

- self-medication, traditional healing, midwifery and the sale of modern drugs.
- work of village health workers (VHWs) and village health committees (VHCs), and all related activities of villagers aimed at enhancing community health, such as a joint drugs fund or an effort to construct and maintain a community water supply system.
- outreach activities of the BHS, with regard to e.g. immunisation or family planning.

None of the three categories is, of course, self-contained; there is continuous interaction. Examples of interaction are the training of traditional midwives in hygienic practices, supervision of VHWs by the BHS, and the involvement of villagers in the planning of a vaccination campaign.

In a broad sense, the first two categories together may be called community based health care (CBHC). When discussing activities at community level in the context of the PHC approach, as in the present paper, it is useful, however, to limit the CBHC concept to the second category only - to the work of VHWs and VHCs, and to joint activities geared to enhancement of community health. Though all such activities are community based, they did not necessarily originate with the community. On the contrary, the impetus usually comes from outside, from the BHS, which has also initiated the organisational framework. This linkage with the BHS, which continues in the form of support and supervision, will receive considerable attention in the present paper, which attempts to complement the analysis of the interface between CBHC and BHS presented by Van Balen.

In analyzing the dynamics of CBHC and related problems, the focus here will be on rural areas. Geographically, most attention will be paid to Africa, with considerable emphasis on experience in Francophone Africa. The method followed will be inductive: general statements on various topics will be based on PHC experiences brought together from a wide variety of countries and settings.

## The village population

The village population plays a crucial role in CBHC. It must support and actively participate in health-related activities, and provide VHWs and VHCs. It is well-known among health care staff that, from an epidemiological point of view, there are important distinctions within a village community. Some villagers are more at risk from certain diseases than others, and the consequences of becoming ill are more serious for some groups than for others. However, when the role of the community as a primary actor in shaping and sustaining CBHC is at stake, these same health professionals usually pay little attention to differentiation within village society. It is, on the contrary, assumed that within a village there is a collective pursuit of the same interests, based on the same shared norms and values. It is often this assumption of fundamental unity that guides the BHS in introducing and implementing PHC activities.

A closer look at village society, whether in Africa or Asia, provides a picture of at least some, and often considerable, differentiation. A village is composed of different groups, which may be based on geographic origin, ethnic background, or kinship. Moreover, age and gender may be important principles for strict distinctions within village society. Variations in the economic basis of household sustenance lead to socioeconomic stratification. All such distinctions may be reflected in differences in power with regard to decision making and access to common resources. Further, they are often reproduced in variation in values and may well lead to opposition of interests.

The social reality of the differentiated village provides an important explanation for the occurrence of problems in introducing and sustaining PHC at the community level. One may even argue, as do some anthropologists, that in certain cases the extended family, the lineage or the class-based group are better bases in which to anchor long term health-related and other development activities than the community as a whole.

In any case, it will be very helpful for health personnel to do a community assessment in a village or area where PHC is to be initiated and supported. The results should be used in discussing possible solutions and interventions for the problems encountered. Unfortunately, medically-oriented nurses, midwives and doctors are badly prepared to recognise the ways in which social and cultural factors affect the implementation of PHC at village level. Further, they lack the training necessary for such community assessment. Moreover, many have an urban background; and even those who originate from villages may well have become alienated from their home base due to a long sojourn in an urban environment. To enhance the effectiveness of the well-intentioned efforts of BHS staff to support PHC in the villages, it is crucial that they move beyond common assumptions about the fundamental unity of village society to the reality of differentiation and acquire the tools to do a simple community assessment.

In Africa village health committees (VHCs), which were established by the BHS when VHWs were introduced in the villages, are the organisational basis of CBHC. Elsewhere, as in India, health-related tasks were assigned to existing village councils. Proper training for the VHCs, which have responsibility for supporting VHWs and organising collective action for health promotion has, however, often been lacking. When VHCs were to be elected, this was seldom thoroughly discussed with the community in advance. Consequently, much remained unclear concerning the persons to be elected to the VHC, including the selection criteria (number, gender, age etc.); their tasks and responsibilities regarding enhancement of the health situation; and their relation to the VHW (frequency and content of support and control). In addition, the creation of a VHC, particularly in Francophone Africa, is not the only change in the village administrative structure. Not only health but also other sectors set up village committees to further their policies at this level. It is not uncommon to witness two or three committee meetings in the same village in one day, e.g. on water, agricultural extension, and health; they compete for time, money and resources. But in any case, creating new village-level organisational structures or - without sufficient discussion, training and guidance - adding to the existing tasks and responsibilities, does not exactly provide conditions conducive to motivation and perseverance of the people involved. Not surprisingly, in the course of time VHCs may grow inactive due to disillusionment on the part of their members, and village councils may concentrate on more familiar tasks. Only more and timely preparatory discussion with villagers and, probably, additional organisational skills among BHS staff will make it possible to build the necessary organisational framework for CBHC.

There is another important aspect of the organisational side of CBHC. Each village has its leadership structures, sometimes including a village council, which reflect balances of power between kinship groups, classes, sexes and generations. As demonstrated in the 1960s, the boomtime of community development policies, newly introduced committees and councils will reflect these existing balances of power.

Specific action and perseverance are therefore required to build organisational structures that provide channels for the less powerful, such as women, the young and the economically weak, to enhance their chances of health improvement. Such efforts will go beyond the straightforward establishment of a VHC. The outsiders involved in the process of introduction - in this case BHS staff - will need to be able and prepared to support rather far-reaching institutional changes in the villages, and to tactfully confront those who resist anything they consider a threat to the existing situation. Here it will become clear that the role of BHS staff in supporting CBHC, as seen from the village perspective, may have strong political aspects; in realising PHC, this implies one more constraint.

### Village health workers

In Africa, village level health workers are generally of two types:

- the young, male and literate VHW, trained in curative and preventive work (here referred to as the VHW, unless stated otherwise); and
- the elderly, illiterate female traditional birth attendant (TBA), who deals with childbirth.

The VHW is chosen by the villagers on the basis of a variety of selection criteria: candidates should, for instance, be permanent residents, have the people's confidence, and be able to read and write. In reality, however, the selection process often is such that major factions within the village community compete regarding the few candidates to finally be appointed by the village chief, with minimal internal consultation and discussion. Unless it is an explicit part of the BHS's approach to the village community, this process often happens almost invisibly, and can scarcely be influenced by the BHS staff, as this decision remains within the realm of the VHC. (See also the extensive description given by Bentley in Chapter 6 of VHWs in Somalia, Eastern Africa.)

There is a major difference between the VHW and the TBA. The TBA is, in fact, an existing institution within village society, including traditional modes of operation and ways of reward and support. The VHW, on the contrary, is a new concept that comes from outside; it is not yet embedded in the existing social structure. After several weeks training (by nurse, midwife and/or doctor) in a district or subdistrict health centre, both will go back to their village, the TBA with a kit containing the material necessary for a clean delivery, and the VHW with the 10-15 essential drugs for treating the most common ailments in the community. How the kits are to be replenished has often not been discussed in detail with the community, the VHC or even with the VHWs/TBAs themselves.

It is not by chance that VHWs in Francophone Africa are usually educated youth. It has, in fact, always been assumed that VHWs should be literate. BHS staff have not been prepared to adapt their training procedures and data collection systems to the needs and abilities of illiterate VHWs. Besides, it has been assumed that handling drugs can only be done by literate people. The BHS set the tone for the current composition of the VHW corps accordingly: young males, since elderly men and most women lag far behind in educational status and writing capability. To the extent that the position of VHW is a coveted resource in a village, it is further to be expected that the young men selected will belong to the most powerful lineage or faction.

There are, however, also countries, such as Botswana, where many VHWs are female, and often not very young. However, it is difficult to find women with an adequate educational level. Permanence of residence may also be a problematic requirement, since in patrilineal societies women tend to leave their village of origin when they marry, but to return there permanently when they are widowed or divorced. Moreover, a VHW position is economically not very attractive to many women, who instead often prefer to spend as much time as possible working the land.

In the course of time the initial tasks and functions of the VHW have gradually increased. Once the concept of a VHW (chosen, controlled and financially supported by the villagers) was accepted by the BHS, they tended to endow the VHW with additional tasks and responsibilities, usually without taking local needs as a guiding concept. Thus, we may observe a VHW performing his regular curative and preventive tasks, keeping track of vital statistics in the village, doing TB case detection and leprosy control, participating in regular weighing sessions for nutritional surveillance, and, when required by BHS staff, organising and preparing vaccination sessions during the visit of the EPI (Expanded Programme on Immunisation) team. Their workload has gradually been extended to a level that they cannot realistically be expected to carry out in a qualitatively acceptable way.

Nevertheless, we cannot expect the VHC or the VHW to draw the line: they are part of a PHC system that takes for granted that BHS staff set the rules. Besides, the addition of new tasks makes the job a more prestigious one. But at the same time, all these tasks defined by the BHS often make the VHW an 'extension worker', who has become alienated from his village population. Conflicts occur between VHC and VHW when it becomes unclear on whose side the VHW is operating.

## The role of the BHS

Putting the blame for problems in CBHC entirely on the basic health services, however, is too easy. There are some good reasons why the contributions of the BHS staff to a well-functioning and effective CBHC have not materialised.

Within the BHS there was, in fact, hardly any experience or familiarity with a methodology for working together with a village community. It was eight years after Alma-Ata before CESAO (the Centre for Economic and Social Studies of West Africa) in Burkina Faso published a manual on 'how to implement PHC at the village level' for Francophone Africa. A similar book for Anglophone Africa, including both medical needs and social and cultural variables to be taken into account at the paramedical level, does not yet exist, to the best of our knowledge. Thus in general BHS staff were working, as it were, in a vacuum, trying to reach certain objectives on the basis of prevailing assumptions.

Two of these assumptions, the need for VHWs to be literate and the view of village society as a unity, have already been mentioned. Others concern the remuneration of VHWs and the payment structure for drugs, which will be discussed below. The fact that the BHS staff consists of medical doctors and nurses who receive no training in social science and are not familiar with the kind of support this discipline can provide has precluded the possibility of going beyond such assumptions and developing intervention methodologies. One such methodology involves establishing a kind of deal or 'contract' between BHS and villagers, spelling out the rights and obligations on each side. Such an approach is of course only feasible on the basis of equal partnership and mutual trust. But often the village is considered too ignorant to participate in such a deal, while among the villagers a feeling of 'wait and see' has prevailed.

*BHS and other providers*

In many countries PHC is the domain of health departments. Government bureaucracies look for easily manageable and replicable interventions and aim at large scale application of principles that seem feasible. However, they often lack the motivation, vision and perseverance necessary to allow for flexible and adaptive PHC implementation.

If non-governmental organisations (NGOs), which in some regions like Anglophone Africa generally come in the form of missions, but elsewhere are often secular organisations, are engaged in promoting PHC, there is often more room for bottom-up approaches. Situational analysis and rapid appraisal techniques may then be used to determine realistic and affordable solutions to health problems together with the village population. The organisational flexibility required to implement the methodology suggested above, in which a 'contract' is made between BHS and villagers, may also be more readily available.

In fact, some NGO projects, e.g. Gono Shasthaya Kendra in Bangladesh and Jamkhed in India, are well-known testing grounds where innovative CBHC approaches have been developed. The extensive PHC programmes that are being promoted by Indian state governments have been influenced by the work of NGOs. In other South Asian countries, e.g. Bangladesh and Pakistan, CBHC as a component of government PHC programmes has barely gotten off the ground. One reason is the many sources of modern Western medicine are already present at village level in the form of drug shops and unlicensed medical practitioners. In such environments VHWs with primarily preventive tasks and few curative skills and medicines - the services villagers usually ask for - cannot successfully compete.

**The issue of VHW remuneration**

A major issue with regard to the continuity of CBHC is whether the services of the VHW ought to be rewarded, and if so, how. Experience shows a range of available options:
• the VHW is paid regularly, for instance monthly, by the government, through the BHS. This alternative has been chosen in, for instance, Liberia, Zimbabwe, and India. In the long run it is, however, hardly feasible for many governments to pursue this policy as economic recession, the restrictions of structural adjustment, and the debt crisis interfere with spending for service delivery.
• the VHW receives no payment from the BHS, but is remunerated in cash or in kind by the community. This alternative may take several forms:

a. the VHW is paid by the VHC from collective village income, as is the case in the cotton producing zone in South Mali;

b. the VHW is allowed to add a small service charge to the price of the drugs he sells. This makes him, in fact, a small medical entrepreneur. Monopolisation of knowledge and skills by the VHW is more likely to occur, as collective financial control is lacking. Only a limited number of VHWs can be active per village, to guarantee a minimum cash income for each VHW. This income is perceived by the VHW more as 'pocket money' than as a 'salary' for his work;

c. alternately, the amount of the surcharge may be controlled by the government. Niger initially allowed a controlled profit on drug sales at village level;

d. the management of the money earned through sale of drugs may be the mutual responsibility of the BHS, together with representatives of the community. This is the case in Pahou, Benin, where part of the income from the sales of drugs is returned to the VHW by a Communal Health Committee as a fixed monthly income.
• the VHW works without payment in cash or kind, as a volunteer. This option is only feasible under specific conditions:

a. if the number of VHWs is increased, to diminish the workload of each individual VHW and to avoid the already mentioned 'monopolisation of knowledge'. This option has been put into effect in Guinea-Bissau. A special variant is to add female VHWs to the already operational male VHWs, as has been tried in the Ségou region of Mali as a means of lowering the threshold for women and children, who often under-utilise the male VHW;

b. if the VHC actively supports the tasks of the VHWs and in this way lightens their workload, as is the case in San (Mali);

c. a more active role of the VHC is also possible if the size of the VHC is increased and each individual member becomes responsible for a limited number of households. This again lightens the workload of the VHW. This alternative has been documented in Gakpé/Pahou, Benin, and in the north of that country, in the Atacora. There, each member of the VHC (family health worker) has a limited number of tasks to perform for members of his homestead or family.

It is important that the staff of the BHS discuss these alternatives with the villagers, so that the community can make an 'informed decision' on how to guarantee the continuity of CBHC. That is, serious attention must be paid to the remuneration issue, taking the existing social structure into account.

Moreover, a decision must be taken within the health department regarding payment of persons referred to the BHS by the VHW. In line with the principle of continuity of care, villagers who contribute to the remuneration of the VHW should be allowed curative care at the BHS without an additional charge. In this way the BHS, in fact, officially recognises the activities of the VHW as the lowest rung of the health care pyramid.

## Preconditions for viable CBHC

Realisation of viable CBHC, which will continue for many years at an acceptable level of quality and with extensive coverage, presupposes that a number of preconditions have been met. Some of these have already been discussed above. It seems worthwhile, however, to list these preconditions as completely as possible, as a recognition of the practical lessons learned since Alma-Ata.

- In its best form, CBHC is tailored to its specific social and cultural context. This means, for instance, that all segments of society should be represented in the VHC. It also means that people's ideas and beliefs regarding the origin and cure of certain diseases and the concomitant health-seeking behaviour must be taken into account when CBHC is taking shape. We should also not forget that CBHC is not new: traditional healers and drug sellers have been practicing it for a long time. Their activities and the self-medication practices that are part of the village culture belong to the environment with which CBHC, in the narrow sense we have been discussing, must be in balance.
- Tailoring PHC to its specific context implies that a 'blueprint' approach to CBHC implementation is always self-defeating. Taking the elementary PHC principles as a guide, in each case the most suitable form of CBHC must be found and realised. This can only be done through a process that includes community assessment, learning by doing, discussions with villagers, creation of broad village support, and adaptation of activities to local conditions.
- Though initial outside support from donors may seem to be a great help, in the long run external financial support - apart from training inputs - is usually self-defeating.

Donors always want a say in what they support, and after a start-up period they will be reluctant to pay recurrent costs for a project or programme. These are two good reasons to be prudent when donors seek to support CBHC, as they are often an impediment to the development of real self-reliance. Conditions attached to donor support should therefore be analysed and discussed before proposals are submitted.

- The continuity of CBHC is closely related to finding an adequate answer to the question of whether to financially reward VHWs, and if so, how. This also implies arriving at a proper definition of the base for their work: the village, the household or the individual. In other words, should the VHW be rewarded by the whole village on a collective or individual basis or should more VHWs per village be trained, thus avoiding cumbersome financial transactions at village level. As noted above, another possibility is to have the VHW supported by a group of households, e.g. those belonging to one lineage, with which the VHW has a special relationship.
- In the selection of VHWs, the issues of literacy, gender and age should be carefully addressed. Experience indicates that mature illiterate VHWs often function better and with more sense of responsibility than many of their younger, literate colleagues. This may, of course, imply that the BHS will have to make an effort to find creative solutions when the illiteracy of VHWs who have been selected precludes their full participation in CBHC activities.
- The composition of the VHC should adequately reflect the heterogeneity of village society, and particular attention should be given to the representation of vulnerable groups such as women and the poor. Furthermore, the members of the VHC must have the leadership and management qualities necessary to keep the committee together and working as an efficient and effective structure. If there are additional committees with development objectives in a village, integrating them will probably contribute to their cohesion and effectiveness.
- CBHC can only be successful if the participating parties act according to the rules. Hence, the rules must be clear, and the issue of accountability must be discussed and its operation defined. The parties involved, i.e. primarily the BHS and the villagers, should preferably work towards a 'deal' on the specifics of CBHC in their special situation. Such a deal should spell out duties (e.g. with regard to the training and supervisory support to be provided by the BHS and the payments to be given to VHWs by the villagers) and rules regulating the referral of patients. But it must also establish a modus for regular discussions between the parties, to guarantee accountability and, if needed, adaptation of the rules to changing conditions.

The above remarks regarding the nature of CBHC and the suggestions as to its operation are based on practical experience, but these are, of course, limited in scope and nature. Other solutions to prevailing problems may have been found elsewhere, or tried and ultimately discarded. It is essential that BHS staff who are involved in the formulation and implementation of CBHC keep an open mind when looking for solutions most suitable to their specific conditions. This implies that notions which are more or less taken for granted, like the position of VHWs as a cornerstone of CBHC, should always be discussable.

Chapter 4

# Personnel development and training

*Fred Abbatt*

Primary Health Care is about people and their interactions. Thus the quality of PHC depends very much on the calibre of the people who provide PHC and the way they interact with the people they serve. Therefore, from this human point of view, the way health care personnel are trained and the ways their capacity to provide health care continues to be developed is of fundamental importance to PHC.

Economic implications also point up the importance of personnel development. Most health care systems spend about 70 to 80 per cent of their budgets directly on labour costs. Within the PHC part of a health system, the proportion may be even higher. If health care personnel work at less than their full potential, the possible wastage of resources can be very high indeed. To illustrate this point, in some studies the gap between actual performance and potential is more than 70 per cent - thus more than half the resources spent on health are in effect wasted. This is obviously of very great significance, especially in those countries where resources are most limited.

Whilst personnel development and training are obvious fields in which action can be taken to improve the quality of PHC, it must be remembered that health care workers do work within a system. This system may impose constraints: unhelpful regulations on working practice or lack of necessary equipment, drugs or facilities. Further, the system may have a powerful effect due to less easily specified factors such as ethos, rewards system and general morale, which will all affect the way health workers carry out their work. So, whilst personnel development and training are of great importance, they are not the only issues which influence quality of health care.

The following sections will review the progress made to date in training personnel for PHC, and then identify some priorities for future action.

## Alma-Ata to the present day

This section presents a series of issues in personnel development and training, considering for each one first the situation at the time of Alma-Ata, then comparing with the present day and identifying aspects where improvements are most urgent. This review is so general that exceptions to almost any statement could be found. However, the review represents the widespread experience of a number of people in many developing countries.

*Numbers and cadres of health workers*

Over the past ten years remarkable changes have taken place in health personnel; perhaps the most obvious is the dramatic increase in the number and diversity of cadres. Ten years ago many countries perceived that they suffered from a serious shortage of doctors; at that time there were enormous increases in the number of medical schools and the number of medical students at each school. This expansion has led in many countries to satisfaction of the perceived need for doctors and to the exhaustion of countries' capacity to employ more doctors, so that unemployment amongst doctors is now a serious concern. Few countries now see a need to expand their training programmes for doctors, and some are reducing medical school intakes.

Just at the time the number of doctors being trained was rapidly expanding, the variety of health worker cadres changed dramatically, although both these changes began prior to the Alma-Ata declaration. Medical assistants, health assistants, village health workers, community health workers etc. appeared in profusion. In general, job descriptions for these new cadres placed increased emphasis on health promotion and the prevention of disease, though curative care was not neglected. Job descriptions were often quite restricted; thus the principle that even if a health worker had been successfully trained, she/he could not be expected to carry out all health care functions, but only those previously defined, became more firmly established. Nevertheless the tendency was to train personnel for a comprehensive role, rather than for a single purpose such as malaria control. The new health care workers thus often had responsibilities in many different aspects of health care, but were deliberately restricted in the depth of the services they were allowed or expected to provide.

As a consequence of this approach it was possible to train health workers with relatively little prior education; indeed many trainee health workers were unable to read or write. Further, the duration of training was often severely restricted, sometimes being only a few months or even weeks. To achieve the maximum benefit from this short training period, innovative course structures were devised and in curriculum design much more attention was paid to task analysis.

As for doctors, the number trained exploded, and here too the capacity of health systems to employ the new cadres of health workers have been exhausted in many countries. The expansion phase is generally over, or coming to an end.

In summary, the dramatic expansion in the absolute number of health workers employed that has taken place in most countries is now complete or approaching completion. Similarly, the variety of cadres of stable health workers has also increased rapidly, but seems unlikely to increase much further over the next decade.

*Learning objectives of training programmes*

The introduction of new cadres of health workers provided opportunities to design training programmes that were not inhibited by tradition or precedent. In many cases this opportunity was accepted and the concepts of 'competency-based curricula' and 'task-oriented curricula' were introduced. Where this was done, training programmes developed away from the traditional medical disciplines that had dominated medical schools, so that the newly designed training programmes were more closely related to the work health workers would be doing.

This trend was reflected in medical schools, but usually only to a limited extent. For example, more attention was paid to behavioral sciences, and 'community health' was given greater, but still very limited, emphasis. A network of community based medical schools was established internationally, but to date only a tiny proportion of all the medical schools have joined, and the extent to which graduates of these medical schools really are different to the graduates of other medical schools is open to question.

The real development therefore has been in the training of the newer cadres of health worker, perhaps especially where this training has been designed and implemented by non-governmental organisations. (Also see Dueñas, Nangawe and Bentley regarding training.) For example, some organisations have used workshops for current health workers to define the tasks they currently carry out, and have then gone on to use this list of tasks as the basis for a new training curriculum.

Whilst the concept of basing curricula on an analysis of tasks appears to have become quite widely accepted, the extent of implementation of this concept remains disappointing. It is still too common to find that learning objectives in practice pay too much attention to memorising medical facts and too little to attitudes, to communication skills and to the performance of health care tasks. Looked at in another way, the emphasis in learning objectives is still too much related to the cure of sick people and the treatment of disease, rather than to disease prevention, health promotion and the management of health care services. In short, despite significant changes, learning objectives have still not taken sufficient account of the extent to which PHC is different from conventional medical care.

*Teaching methods*

At the time of Alma-Ata, medical education exhibited some of the best practice in higher education in the teaching methods used. Medical schools were among the leaders in the application of the then current educational technology, which was very much equipment based. In general this was a response to the priorities of the time, how to maintain quality in the face of rapidly expanding student numbers with little corresponding increase in numbers of teachers. Thus substantial developments took place in the use of film, television, 35 mm slides, audio tapes etc. Elegant systems for students to use self-learning packages in teaching laboratories were introduced and computer-based learning was becoming important. However, these developments had two major deficiencies. Their expense and technical complexity meant they could only be applied in situations with substantial financial and technical resources, so they had little impact in poorer countries or in training less prestigious cadres of health workers. Second, the technology generally focused on more effective transmission of information; it did not do much to stimulate the student to respond to or process the information. Thus the educational technology of the time did little to support the need for students to achieve new objectives; it merely helped them achieve the old objectives more efficiently.

During the past ten years there has been an important shift of emphasis in teaching methodology, especially in training lower cadres of health personnel. Teaching methods now emphasise using smaller groups in discussion and project work, more time is spent in the field and in work with communities. More effort is made to organise practical work and to develop health care skills through simulation and games.

However, despite significant progress it is still true that teachers generally rely too heavily on lecturing and presenting facts. Sometimes this is done deliberately, openly and consciously. At other times teachers may claim to be using more sophisticated and appropriate techniques, but in practice spend much of their time presenting information in a slightly modified lecture style.

*Teaching materials*

One of the immediate problems faced by the teachers of PHC workers at the time of Alma-Ata was that very few appropriate teaching materials existed. What was available tended to be at too high a level (intended for doctors or sometimes nurses), written in English or other European languages, related to curative care in developed countries and only available from developed country publishers, and therefore requiring hard currency. Since that time, much has been achieved. The WHO Programme on Health Learning Materials, Teaching Aids at Low Costs (TALC), African Medical and Research Foundation (AMREF), and many other groups and organisations, have done much to make available materials related to local health problems. These are more appropriate for the cadres of health personnel to be trained and are produced in the developing world at reasonable cost. A network for Francophone countries is now being created.

Despite the very substantial achievements, there is still much to be done. This is partly a question of quantities of materials required for distribution to all health workers or all students. Partly it is a question of quality; many materials are poorly written and designed, so that the intended audience has very great difficulty reading and using the materials. Partly it is a question of relevance; the main emphasis of much teaching material is still on the conventional medical disciplines and on curative care. Very little on effective and feasible techniques related to health promotion, communication skills, community participation and the management of health care on a community basis is available that is practical and relevant.

*Assessment*

The assessment methods used during and at the end of training programmes are of enormous importance in shaping what trainees actually learn; trainees naturally attempt to master the skills that will be tested during in-course or end of course examinations or assessments. Further, assessment if well done can provide feedback on the success of training and thus input for planning future training programmes.

At the time of Alma-Ata there was a trend towards increased use of in-course assessment and also towards more objective methods of assessment such as multiple choice questions. Even so, much of the assessment of health workers still depended heavily on final exams consisting of essay questions or short practical/clinical tests.

Since Alma-Ata, the opportunities provided by the need to design new curricula for new cadres of health workers have been exploited to ensure increased emphasis on in-course assessment and objective assessment methods. There have also been a number of attempts to broaden the range of skills tested through techniques such as the Objective Structured Clinical Examination (OSCE). However, these worthwhile developments remain insufficient to fully reflect the changes in health care that are implicit in PHC policies. Medical schools, with a few exceptions, still virtually ignore the assessment of skills other than those directly related to the diagnosis and treatment of individual patients. For other cadres more attention is paid to preventive aspects, yet too little is done to assess e.g. communication and management skills. Hence assessments rarely provide a valid test of the skills needed for successful PHC. Further, assessment systems are commonly unreliable: the marks awarded correlate only weakly with the actual skill of the students assessed.

*In-service training*

In 1987 in-service training or continuing education was generally only a matter of concern to doctors, and to a much lesser extent hospital nurses. Most newer cadres had been in existence for such a short time that their initial training was often very recent; there was as yet little need for 'refresher training'. But although continuing medical education was by comparison much commoner, there were already significant concerns about its value. Literature reviews in North America showed little evidence that continuing medical education had any impact on the provision of health care.

Since Alma-Ata, a number of factors have focused attention on the need for in-service training for all PHC workers. These factors include the realisation that the relative isolation of many PHC workers means they have little peer contact through which they can learn and maintain morale. Secondly, the quality of the health care and supervision provided has been questioned; in-service education has been seen as offering some solution. Thirdly, as new techniques have become available, in-service training has been seen as the appropriate method of introducing these techniques throughout the work force. Fourthly, donor agencies have regarded in-service training as a legitimate and appropriate way of providing aid, and as one of the few methods from which a high rate of implementation can be expected.

For all these reasons, in-service training has become much more common throughout the whole range of health care workers, receiving substantial resources of finance and time. However, it should not be simply assumed that benefits will be obtained. Whilst undoubtedly there are potentially very substantial benefits to be expected from effective in-service training, which are often obtained, there remain too many examples of in-service training that is so poorly designed or implemented that the benefit is negligible.

Some of the problems associated with less effective in-service training result from the organisational structure that decides the type of training. This decision is usually made at national level, and may be a response to external donor agencies. Whilst this is not harmful in itself, it does present the danger that several uncoordinated training activities may take place at similar times, burdening the health worker in the field with unrealistic expectations for change in too many different aspects of his/her work. Secondly, the educational design often pays far too little attention to the psychology of innovation and the principles of adult learning. As a result, information may be transmitted to the trainee, but not be accepted and incorporated into new work patterns.

The end result of these and other problems is that the organisers' high expectations of in-service training are rarely realised. Participants too often have high expectations of something generally worthwhile, but may not expect something that leads to changes in the way they work.

*Organisation and systems*

The various achievements and shortcomings of the past decade can be traced back to the organisational structures and systems that have made the achievements possible and the shortcomings probable.

First, Ministries of Health and NGOs have accepted PHC policies, and in many cases have established units or departments responsible for implementing these policies. This has made possible the introduction of the new cadres of health worker. There has also been a major expansion in the number and size of educational institutions, which has made possible the training of very much larger numbers of health workers.

However, in many countries there is little that could be called a human resources system. Such a system would take into account national resources and policies for health, together with an analysis of health-related needs, and use these to derive job descriptions for the work to be done in health care. These job descriptions would define the work to be done by each cadre of health personnel and so provide clear and precise objectives for each training programme in terms of numbers of people to be trained and what they should learn. This in turn would define what is taught and, crucially, what is assessed during the training programme.

This simple concept of a human resources system is extremely difficult to implement in practice, because it requires a high degree of coordination between people who have conventionally seen their responsibilities as separate and independent. For example, health care managers at district level have rarely been regarded as appropriate people to serve as examiners in training institutions for health personnel; yet these are the people who should know best what standard of performance is required. (In situations where community participation is highly developed, 'managers' may include lay members of the community.) A less controversial example relates to the number of people trained. Surprisingly often Ministries of Health have little information available about the number and ages of people currently employed in each cadre of health personnel. Nor do they have reliable information about numbers leaving service for various reasons. Thus it is difficult to predict the number who should be accepted for training. On the other hand, when this information is available it may not be acted upon, because training institutions take pride in their independence and therefore are unwilling to accept limits on students entry imposed by 'others'.

These are only examples. Many instances could be used to illustrate the lack, or at least the weakness, of the human resources system for health personnel.

Another aspect of the organisational structure that has fundamental effects is the career structure of teachers of health workers. Two major problems can occur. First, entry qualifications for the profession of teaching health workers commonly ignore the need for competence in teaching; teachers are often appointed solely on the basis of health care qualifications. Indeed there are remarkably few opportunities for teachers to receive training in teaching skills. As a result, teaching health workers is an intrinsically amateur profession - with the predictable consequence that whilst some of the teachers do have great natural talent and do develop their skills by learning from experience, there remain a substantial number whose technical competence in teaching skills is extremely limited.

The second problem regarding the career structure is that for many teachers there is very little prospect of promotion. In some cases the more senior posts are held by medically qualified personnel and are not open to others with different health care qualifications. Another common situation is that there is very little opportunity for transfer between teaching and field posts. Thus teachers have little contact with the realities of health care in the field, and are also prevented from seeking promotion via transfer to field posts. This situation inevitably affects morale and motivation.

Funding is the final factor in the organisation of personnel development and training to be considered here. In part difficulties here relate to an absolute shortage of resources, and in part to the control of those resources that are available.

Effective training inevitably costs money. Teacher's salaries and accommodation for trainees are usually the major costs. In some countries training costs are minimised by insisting on unrealistic teacher:student ratios, or by providing such unsuitable accommodation for trainees that this interferes with the learning process. However, this is often not the problem. The financial aspect that is most commonly a problem is the size of the budget available for books, paper, teaching materials, and transport. Economies in these areas of expenditure are particularly unfortunate, since the total proportion of the budget devoted to non-salary/accommodation costs is almost always very small, yet the effect of shortages can be very serious. Shortages in overall funding often become more serious than necessary when control over the way money is spent is highly centralised.

## Priorities for the future

As the outline above indicates, many significant developments in the training of health personnel have occurred in the ten years since Alma-Ata. Yet the quality of health care available in many countries is still seriously restricted - not just by lack of resources, but by inappropriate systems and methods of training for health workers. The following section suggests some priorities for action that would help to make fuller implementation of PHC policies possible over the next decade.

*Developing a human resources system*

A fundamental development that is urgently needed in many countries is an integration of management and training functions for health personnel. This integration might take the form of a reorganisation of government departments such that defining job descriptions, day-to-day management of health workers, and training of health workers all come under a single department of 'human resources'. However, such a reorganisation is unlikely to take place. Mechanisms for coordination between existing departments are the alternative. These will vary from one situation to another, but this is unimportant. The important issue is the quality of the coordination achieved.

Effective coordination will lead to unity of purpose with regard to:

• work to be done by each cadre of health worker. Whilst the balance of work will vary from one community to another, the job description and the detailed methods of working should be precisely defined. This is done for more clinical aspects (e.g. aseptic techniques), but is rarely achieved in health education, community involvement/participation and so forth.

• initial training of health workers. Teaching, learning experiences and assessment should be designed at a minimum to ensure competence in all of the defined aspects of the job description. All (or at least a very high proportion) of the defined skills should be mastered. This need not be restrictive, however, since additional skills and information may also be learnt.

• in-service training of health workers. The in-service training programme should be seen as one way of solving problems in providing health care. That is, in-service training should be seen as a management tool. Thus managers, rather than teachers, will define what needs to be learnt during in-service training.

• supervision of health workers. The frequency and regularity of supervision will often need to be improved. But more important than the number of visits is their nature. The role of the supervisor as a problem-identifier and a problem-solver should be emphasised. Problems may relate to poor quality of work or inadequate resources. Where deficiencies in working methods are identified, the main strategy for improvement should be education, either on a one-to-one basis implemented by the supervisor, or, where problems are common, through some form of group-based in-service training.

• number of health workers to be trained. The number of health workers accepted for training should be based on projections of the number of each cadre to be employed in future years, together with projections for dropouts, retirement and promotion.

*Increasing competence of teachers*

Many of the deficiencies in the training of health workers stem from the limited competence in educational skills of many of their teachers. This is inevitable, since opportunities for acquiring such skills are severely limited. Similarly, the rewards for becoming expert in this profession are often limited: little recognition is usually given the excellent teachers who do exist, and there are few opportunities for promotion. Competence could be increased by:

• establishing centres in every country to train teachers of health workers. (Such centres do exist in a few countries). These centres could also serve as foci for the development of locally relevant and appropriate teaching materials, curricula and even assessment instruments;

• establishing career structures for teachers of health workers, so that excellence can be rewarded by promotion. A substantial period of training in the skills of teaching as a condition of entry to the profession might be one feature of such a career structure;

• providing systematic in-service training in educational methodology for all existing teachers of health workers;
• establishing relations with nursing schools.

*Raising the status of training*

In health care, human resources issues often seem to be neglected in comparison to other more immediate and intellectually accessible issues such as drug supplies, immunisation, or distribution of health resources. As a consequence, health personnel training tends to be low on the political agenda, and sometimes people whose competence is poorly regarded are placed in posts with responsibility for health personnel training since 'they will do the least harm there'. Naturally this is a damaging situation, but it is hard to see how it can be changed. Some possibilities are:
• for donor agencies to place health personnel training higher in their own priorities;
• for governments, together with donor agencies, to take greater advantage of existing opportunities to train Ministry of Health staff in the broader issues of health personnel training (i.e. not just teaching methodology, but management of training systems);
• for some increase of resources to be made available to training institutions, especially those involved in training lower status health personnel. This increase need be, in many countries, only a small percentage of the total budget for health personnel training, provided it is allocated to the provision of teaching/learning materials;
• for international or bilateral agencies to pay much greater attention to human resources systems when conducting national health reviews.

*Strengthening communication/community involvement skills*

The priorities above relate to all training programmes, and can be expected to yield benefits throughout training. However, one whole area of skills is generally poorly learnt: the poorly defined area related to health promotion, community development, community participation etc. This area is especially important: for many health workers this is what makes the work they actually do different from what they would have done under the health care policies that preceded PHC. Ironically it is these very areas of difference that are least well defined and understood. To remedy this situation it will be important to:
• establish a set of techniques in these vaguely defined areas that have been shown to work in the field, so they can be taught to health care workers;
• develop teaching materials and assessment items that are specifically designed to teach these skills, once they have been defined.

For each of the above priorities, the end point of a process has been suggested; little attention has been paid to how this end point may be achieved. Successful achievement will naturally depend on many inputs, from diverse sources. However, donor agencies may well have the key role to play in financing some of the initiatives, providing some of the intellectual leadership that will assist in advocating these priorities, and supporting communication between countries that will help governments and NGOs learn from each other's experiences.

## The need for research

The overall priority in personnel development and training is not for research; it is to implement what is already known and established. However, there are a number of areas where research would be valuable. These include:

- teaching/learning methods for illiterates. Whilst PHC has made significant advances in employing personnel with little or no formal education, rather little is known about the best ways of teaching or assessing such staff during their training periods. Clearly, increased knowledge in these areas could be of enormous practical benefit to the quality of health care less literate people can provide, and to the learners themselves;
- economic benefits of in-service training/supervision. Many of those who provide in-service training or advocate increased and improved supervision believe resources spent on these activities yield commensurate benefits. Yet direct evidence for such benefits is weak, and is rarely expressed in cost-benefit terms. Research is needed to quantify changes in work performance following in-service training or an intensified programme of supervision. The benefits of these changes could be expressed in economic terms and thus could be used to justify future decisions regarding in-service training. Such research, if it pointed to clear economic benefits, would help to refute the arguments of those who believe that in-service training or supervision is a luxury that can only be afforded in wealthier countries;
- techniques of health education/community involvement. Much teaching about health education or community involvement is based either on philosophical grounds (why such activities should be undertaken) or on very limited anecdotal evidence. Therefore there is a need to establish a much more scientific basis for the ways different types of behaviour can be modified through health education, the ways communities can be stimulated to participate in health care, and the ways health workers can encourage community development.

When, and only when, these processes are better understood can teaching programmes be developed that will be more effective in teaching health care workers these important skills.

## Conclusion

Personnel development and training in PHC has made significant advances in the past ten years. Yet the preparation of health workers in such a way that they achieve a higher proportion of their potential for providing health care remains a challenge. In meeting this challenge, the priorities are to integrate the management of health systems much more closely with the training of health workers, so that an effective human resources system is established. This will provide a framework within which existing well established educational techniques can be implemented in an effective manner, thereby helping to achieve health for all by the year 2000.

## Chapter 5

# Financing systems and resource use

*Lucy Gilson*

Health workers and communities have a vital role to play in deciding what changes in financing are desirable and feasible. However, although financing problems undermine the day to day work of every health worker, health financing is generally seen as the preserve of 'the economist'. This chapter is therefore intended to encourage all those involved in health care delivery to think about health financing. The issues that underlie the current health financing debate are set out, and some suggestions are made regarding the approach to adopt in addressing the resource problems of the health sector in a way compatible with the PHC approach.

Affordability is a key facet of this approach. Indeed, some have seen PHC as a 'cheap option' for health care in developing countries. Provision of preventive and basic curative care at lower tiers of the health system are the focus, in part because such care is less expensive and potentially more effective in improving health status than higher-technology hospital care. More broadly, PHC is concerned with alleviation of health inequalities through health care and general development, by means of community participation in both areas. At its core, therefore, is the pursuit of social justice.

Unfortunately, the Alma-Ata declaration coincided with an early phase of world recession, and economic difficulties have constrained the implementation of PHC policies. What was once seen as affordable has been, in practice, beyond the capacity of many countries. A combination of lower economic growth and population increases led to falls in income and consumption per person in many developing countries in the 1970s, followed by an even sharper drop in 1982. Some countries performed better than others: growth in Asia as a whole in the period was over 5%, but by the end of 1984 average gross domestic product per person in Latin America and the Caribbean had fallen back to the level of 1976. The situation in the Sub-Saharan countries remains especially bleak - by 1983 income per person was about 4% below the level of 1970 (Abel-Smit, 1986).

A common response to this economic crisis has been the adoption of 'structural adjustment' policies, as recommended by the International Monetary Fund: curtailing demand, stimulating exports, devaluing currency and cutting public expenditure. As a result, the proportion of public expenditure devoted to health in all low income countries has been halved, from 6.1% in 1972 to 3% in 1982. This contrasts sharply with the nearly 2% increase (to 11.7%) in the proportion allocated to health in industrial countries over the same period.

The impact of resource constraints on health status is difficult to determine, but evidence now becoming available suggests health status is declining in many parts of the world, and that such declines have occurred during the period of economic recession. Costa Rica, for example, is a country where earlier improvements in infant mortality rates have been reversed - and infant mortality actually rose in 1985. Recent surveys from Botswana and Ghana show a downward trend in nutritional status of children, and it is particularly likely that the health status of the rural and peri-urban poor has deteriorated. 'Health for All by the year 2000' is an elusive goal in times of severe economic constraints.

### Implications for financing choices

These complex problems have led to calls for 'sustainability' within the health sector. The implications of these calls are twofold. First, a drive to improve the use of currently available resources, to improve efficiency and achieve greater cost-effectiveness in health activities. Second, a search for new sources of finance for government health activities and for greater cost recovery in the health sector. This search has been spearheaded by international agencies like the World Bank and UNICEF, who have largely had an African focus in recognition of the particular difficulties of this continent. They have called, in the short run, for the introduction of user charges for curative services and for drugs. For the World Bank this is part of a policy reform package that also includes the introduction of insurance or other risk-sharing schemes, more effective use of the non-governmental health sector and decentralisation of governmental health services. UNICEF's Bamako Initiative calls for the establishment of community level revolving funds for drugs, initially to be supported by external assistance but to become self-supporting through cost-recovering drug charges and community management.

If such changes are to be introduced within PHC they must both provide increased resources for PHC and promote the underlying principles of the PHC approach. Financing mechanisms have diverse effects: they may discourage health service utilisation, encourage the use of one provider over another, and/or promote the growth of high-technology hospital care. Some of these changes may not be appropriate from the perspective of PHC, which is not just a set of activities but also, and more importantly, a process of changing people's understanding of ill-health and changing the nature of health care provision. From this perspective, the impact of any financing mechanism on equity and community participation is a particular concern, because these are central to the concern for social justice.

In practice, the choice of health financing will differ among continents because of their very different existing health and financing systems. Health insurance, for example, represents a large part of Latin American health systems, and is being introduced in some Asian countries, but is unimportant in most African countries. 'Free' (no fee) government health care is widely available to all sections of the population in Africa and Asia, but has a smaller role in Latin America. Modern private practitioners are fairly widely available in most areas of Latin American countries, but are often limited to urban areas in African (and some Asian) countries, and traditional healers are more often consulted by the rural populations of Africa and Asia.

## Health financing: current concerns

*Problems undermining change in allocations and performance*

As noted, the calls for 'sustainability' within the health sector emphasise that not only are resources limited, but also they are used inefficiently and inappropriately. From the PHC perspective, there are currently two problems: health resource allocations favour neither PHC priority activities nor the low-income group of the population who are most vulnerable to ill-health. 50 - 60% of all government spending for health activities in many developing countries is directed towards the provision of urban-based hospital care. In Sri Lanka between 1981 and 1986, recurrent government expenditure on community health activities in one district never rose above 18% of total district expenditures (Attanayake and De Silva, 1987). In Ghana, urban facilities currently receive more than 80% of health ministry's budget (Janovsky and Cassels, 1988) and in Peru, although only about one-third of the population live in the Lima region, it captured about half of the national expenditure for patient-related care in 1984. As a result of these differentials it is often not possible to provide even a minimum package of primary level care to the generally low-income rural population, particularly in Africa. Even within urban areas, as in Mexico City, health services are least accessible to the low income, peri-urban population groups (Ward, 1987).

This allocation pattern is partly the result of political pressure from the urban population and from specialist doctors demanding new medical technology. However, it can be exacerbated by financing mechanisms. Health insurance, private or social, is most easily introduced for higher-income employees in the formal sector who live in urban areas: there are often marked inequalities in the quantity of services available to insured and uninsured populations. These differences may be further accentuated by the tendency for health insurance schemes to attract trained personnel away from the government sector. Like private practice, insurance schemes offer a range of rewards that government services cannot match. Both insurance and private practice also promote high-technology care, as demanded by doctors and their patients. On the other hand, fee systems in which fees increase with the level of service may encourage more appropriate patient use of available services. Under such fee systems, local clinics are less likely to be bypassed for hospitals.

Other inefficiencies in the way resources are used in the health sector include: the construction of buildings without ensuring adequate numbers of personnel or stocks of drugs are available to supply them, resulting in the provision of only a limited range of poor quality care; existing buildings being left to deteriorate, rather than being maintained on a regular basis; and the loss of imported drugs (sometimes up to 70%

between delivery to the country and delivery to peripheral health facilities). As a result it may be possible to make substantial savings within existing resource levels. The Malawi ten year plan (1986-95) identifies potential savings within the recurrent budget of its major referral hospital of nearly 33% of the total budget. Studies of the savings achievable within drug supply and distribution systems show economies varying from an average of 10%, due to better drug selection, to 45%, as a result of better drug storage and distribution.

Financing mechanisms may also have an effect on these resource use problems. Where financial incentives to clinicians favour increased prescribing or other medical interventions, greater inefficiencies may result. A Brazilian study reviewing the demand for Caesarian sections has shown that many such operations requested by doctors in private practice are not necessary on medical grounds, but reflect the financial incentives available to these doctors in private practice (Janowitz et al., 1982).

*Underlying causes.* The primary underlying causes of poor resource use are weak management skills, procedures and information systems. There are few trained health administrators in developing countries; the role of district manager usually falls to senior doctors and nurses in the district, whose training does not include basic management skills such as priority setting, costing and budgeting. District managers also suffer from weak support staff; accountants in particular may also be under-skilled.

Although accountants are often the responsibility of central government financial bodies and not the Ministry of Health, poor resource use within the health sector can often be traced to them. Thus their skills, practices and accountability need to be reviewed in order to improve financial management at all levels of the health system. Such improvements are vital to the successful introduction of new financing mechanisms giving greater financial responsibility to health systems (such as fees retained at the point of service delivery).

In particular, a budget and resource allocation procedure that allows for considerable local control over expenditure is necessary - even if central control is retained over resource allocations among geographical areas, major programmes and large institutions. Existing budget systems have often been established as a form of expenditure control and for accounting purposes, not to support planning activities. Budgeting is, therefore, a completely separate activity from planning. (New budgets tend to be based on old ones. Therefore they favour existing allocation patterns and facilities, rather than reflecting new plans and priorities, e.g. PHC). A more flexible system is essential to ensure that PHC priorities are translated into budget allocations, and that those allocations are used as efficiently as possible.

However, the information needed to plan, budget and manage resources effectively is usually absent in the health sector, especially at district level. Existing health information systems tend to generate (infrequently) a mass of health activity information that is consequently rarely used. Such systems rarely identify information priorities (for example, activity data is not presented in a form useful for management, e.g. splitting first visits and re-visits, and identifying visits per episode). Basic cost data (e.g. total cost per contact and drug cost per contact) and other performance indicators (e.g. drug availability and workload) are excluded. Without such information it is difficult for managers to monitor performance of health services in their areas and provide support where needed to improve performance. (See also Harnmeijer on the calculation of recurrent costs, and Bentley and Nangawe on management.)

Personnel management is another specific weakness of the health sector that must be addressed, since staff are the central resource of health systems. Their morale has a vital influence on the quality of care offered, but in many countries morale has been severely undermined. Although salaries and wages represent an increasing proportion of health budgets, inflation has undercut purchasing power. Doctors and nurses increasingly must work two or more jobs just to meet their families' needs. Such difficulties are compounded by the personnel policies and practices of Ministries of Health, such as moving personnel without warning or consultation; ignoring needs of health workers' families and posting mothers, for example, to remote areas; making it difficult for complaints to be heard; denying fringe benefits (such as free housing in remote areas); denying recognition of further training (e.g. salary increments for additional qualifications); or allocating training awards on an arbitrary and unfair basis. All these issues must be addressed to promote better morale among workers, identify non-financial reward systems and reward hard work and commitment. The underlying problem is the failure of governments to recognise the special needs of the health worker, who is not just another civil servant but often works odd hours in difficult conditions.

If these diverse problems are to be addressed effectively, a government-wide effort will be required. The problems and needs of the health sector must be recognised, if it is not to be continually forgotten in the national resource allocation process and if management weaknesses are to be addressed. The health sector alone cannot confront problems whose roots often lie in government structures and processes. However, it can take steps to improve performance - to develop consultative budgeting and planning processes, to strengthen information systems, to develop managerial skills, to ensure that personnel management is more sensitive to personnel needs. Such improvements are necessary to make better use of available resources, to raise the profile of the health sector and to improve the acceptability of the health service in the eyes of the population. Health financing changes should allow, and not oppose, the achievement of these aims.

*The PHC perspective: need for appropriate change*

The PHC approach is underpinned by a concern for social justice and equity. Equity is difficult to define but is concerned with fairness and whether those who most need health care are able to obtain it. Because the way health programmes are financed and provided influences the distribution of benefits, the impact of any new financing system on equity must be assessed to ensure its appropriateness from the PHC perspective. Such assessment is based on who benefits from health care, who pays for it and the links between the two.

Benefit distribution is partly related to access to health care, but only those who take advantage of access and make use of care will actually benefit. Distribution of benefit must, therefore, be assessed and monitored by reviewing health care utilisation patterns. Many factors influence a decision to use health care; utilisation studies indicate that the community's perception of their health needs and the health services available to them is important. Does government health care address felt needs? Even where government health care is appropriate, is it perceived as effective? Do financing systems influence perceptions of acceptability and patterns of utilisation?

The studies available (Gilson, 1988; Musgrove, 1986) suggest that the price of health care can influence use, but that its influence is connected to the perceived quality of care. Important aspects of perceived quality are the time required to obtain care (either negative, because costly, or positive, because it offers an opportunity to socialise), the attitudes of health personnel and the lack of drugs. Community perceptions have also been found to differ among population groups. The least educated, low income groups are least likely to find government health services acceptable and, therefore, are the most likely not to use them. It is not surprising, therefore, that this group is likely to reduce its utilisation most in response to price increases. Neither it is surprising, given the poor perceptions of the quality of government care, that studies have shown utilisation decreases when charges for government care are increased. Financing health care through user fees may not, therefore, be compatible with the PHC approach.

*The community perspective.* Only by understanding the community's perspective can PHC strategies hope to provide acceptable health care. Therefore the PHC approach stresses the need to plan health activities with the community. For example, in PHC strategies decentralisation is not simply a means of improving management but a way of facilitating community involvement in decision making. The Bamako Initiative emphasises community management of the drug funds it seeks to establish, to ensure that the community has the major say regarding the use of the funds raised. However, appropriate procedures and systems are essential if these good intentions are to be put into practice.

Community financing schemes, in which a community acts to introduce specific health financing mechanisms within their local area, have been one vehicle for community participation in PHC projects over many years. Experience with such schemes suggests the following conclusions about acceptable service delivery and financing patterns:

- community residents are willing to cooperate with each other and with representatives of the health system, if they get high quality goods and services of the type they want;
- this willingness may even extend to relatively unattractive preventive activities, if these are linked to high demand curative care, water supply, income generation, or credit;
- hopes that community financing will be easy because of the large sums that communities are already paying for health are illusory;
- health professionals may be reluctant to countenance compromises in technical quality and equity;
- community financing should not be encouraged if the required level of effort cannot be invested;

• community decision making and management are critical for the sustainability of community based projects.

*A Zairean example.* One specific example of community financing comes from the Belgian-supported Kasongo project in Zaire, which has developed a strategy for financing and providing health care in collaboration with the community. Strong emphasis is given to provision of adequate care, both at the primary and referral levels, and to the development of district level management capacity.

The system is partly self-financed, not only because health sector resources are constrained, but also because self-financing, if properly designed, is believed to promote participatory decision making, adaptation of services to the needs of the community, and a sense of responsibility within the population. Community resources are used to support the health facilities most accessible to and understood by the community, i.e., the primary facility. However, the community cannot meet the full costs of health services; continuing financial support from national or international resources is required.

There are four criteria for choosing a method of self financing: it must contribute to continuity of care (no financial barriers to repeat visits for the same illness episode), it must promote solidarity (fee levels are not based on the cost of care, and the chronically ill pay the same as those less severely ill), it should foster a sense of responsibility in the users of the service (by making them aware of the cost of the care they use, and discouraging unnecessary use of higher levels of care), and it should enable the health system to be financially viable (meet the costs not covered by government). The choice of payment methods is between payment by item of service and a flat rate, periodically paid by each community member or household.

Although this system is based on strong community participation and the provision of good quality care, problems remain. Community resources are inadequate to support entire health systems and complementary funding is still required. The financing creates a pull towards provision of curative care, because this is what the community most demands, not preventive care. Even more important, from the PHC perspective, is that the flexibility inherent in the approach implies an unequal development of regions and a strong likelihood that richer (urban) communities will benefit, both from the existence of government supported hospitals and from their greater capacity to raise resources for health care.

Unless government has both the financial and administrative capacity to counterbalance these trends, differences in health provisions between regions are likely. Even within a community, inequities may be exacerbated if the system is not tailored to the most vulnerable and if it introduces alien and impractical mechanisms into society. For example, payment for health care may traditionally be made in kind (a chicken or grain), but payment for Western systems requires cash (e.g. to buy drugs), which is much less available within subsistence and informal societies. Community participation in decision making may not prevent such problems if the most vulnerable have no voice in the decisions and if the system is determined more by its own needs than those of the community.

*Additional design considerations.* In designing health financing schemes, it is also important to learn more about existing health care payment patterns and community support systems. For example, in Sudan patients may pay traditional healers in kind over a period of time; they are charged according to an informal assessment of income level. The burden of payment is not placed on the individual patient, but on their family, and may be even shared within the wider community. Questions to ask in other communities include: What is the nature of payments made? What is the timing of payments? Who pays for traditional health care? How is support shared within the community? Once this information is gathered, ways must be sought to translate these lessons into practice within more formal systems.

Design of financing mechanisms compatible with the PHC approach must begin with consideration of their impact on equity, and must recognise their potential impact on the acceptability of health care and utilisation patterns. By involving the community in the development of new approaches to financing, it is possible to design mechanisms that are acceptable. However, equity problems may still not be completely resolved.

*The current health financing debate*

Discussion of the potential for addressing the resource problems of the health sector through changes in national financing systems has been led by international agencies. Given the influence of these agencies on national policy making, it is important to examine their arguments.

Both the World Bank and UNICEF base their arguments on the general situation of a country with a predominantly tax-financed and 'free' (no price) government health system, suffering from the inefficiencies in resource use - including inequitable access to health care - faced by most health systems. Financing system changes are required, they suggest, to address these problems. The financing systems they propose are based on the assumption that existing payments for health care represent a willingness to pay for government care and, beyond that, an ability to pay among most population groups. It is, therefore, desirable to capture those household resources now spent on non-government care for the government health service, by levying charges.

The World Bank suggests government responsibility for provision of health care should largely be limited to providing services like immunisation, control of vector-borne diseases, sanitary waste disposal and health education that benefit the community as a whole by preventing the spread of disease. Curative services that benefit only the individuals using them (and have few or no external benefits for the community) should be the responsibility of a combination of non-government (both commercial and non-commercial) and government services. It appears that in Latin America, where non-government curative care is more widespread throughout countries, the government's role in the provision of curative care is envisaged as very small; but in African countries where there are few alternative health providers giving 'effective' care, particularly in rural areas, it is suggested that government will continue to provide a combination of preventive and basic curative services. Such a division of responsibilities is, finally, assumed to permit a diversion of government resources from curative services to preventive services. These programmes (for example, UNICEF stresses maternal and child health programmes) can then be strengthened and extended with the additional resources.

*Failure to address relevant issues.* Although the arguments seem appealing and appear to represent a pragmatic response to the resource problems of the health sector, these proposals do not address the basic causes of inefficiency: political influence over resource allocation decisions, poor management and poor health sector performance. The World Bank calls for service providers to be involved in decisions about the use of additional revenues, to ensure better resource use. However, the introduction of user fees cannot address the lack of management skills and procedures within health systems that underlie poor resource use. Moreover, although fees may encourage more efficient use of service levels by patients, they may encourage inefficient provider behaviours as well.

A further problem is that these proposals are not wholly compatible with the PHC approach and its emphasis on equity and community participation. As discussed, equity is in part related to the use made of health care. Although the price of health care is not always the dominant factor determining use, increasing fees is likely to reduce use, especially by the low income. Willingness to pay cannot, therefore, be assumed to be equivalent to ability to pay - especially for the most vulnerable section of the population and in low income countries, only a small proportion of the total population is apt to be able to afford charges above a very minimal level. In theory it may be possible to protect low income groups from the full burden of charges via an exemption mechanism, perhaps a sliding scale for different income groups. However, experience with exemption mechanisms is limited; the key difficulties relate to the problems of income assessment. How is income to be assessed when much of it is generated through subsistence farming or informal sector business? Who collects the fees and assesses income? How is abuse of the system restricted?

The proposals of the international agencies are also likely to exacerbate equity problems because they are intended as national schemes, initiated not by communities and not even, in some cases, by central governments. Rather than working within communities on a small-scale and gradual basis (as in Zaire) countries have rapidly introduced national fee structures (e.g. Ghana) or have been asked to introduce nation-wide programmes of drug revolving funds (the Bamako Initiative). The community's role in decision making is, therefore, not clear; as a result other efforts at encouraging community participation in primary health care programmes may be undermined.

Why, given these many unresolved questions and the failure of fee systems to address the underlying problems of health systems, do such schemes continue to be promoted? Although difficult to prove, it appears that the international agencies have priorities other than the resolution of health sector financial problems, and that the call for user charges, in particular, reflects a broader approach to economic policy-making.

It is possible to see the roots of the World Bank's call for user charges in a report on the world economic situation published in 1982, which criticised the over-expansion of the state in African countries, as demonstrated by the provision without charge of education, health, and water supply facilities. User charges, therefore, fit neatly into the package of structural adjustment policies recommended by the International Monetary Fund that has been considered/introduced by countries as diverse as Ghana, Mozambique, Tanzania and Uganda. The emphasis underlying this approach is on freeing the market from government intervention and so allowing it to function efficiently: efficiency is seen as the key to improvements in the broad national economic situation as well in the health sector. Change in financing systems is being demanded not simply because of the current difficulties but because the alternative is deemed to be better. However, this assessment of what is 'best' is fundamentally at odds with the PHC approach and especially its emphasis on equity, community participation and the gradual resolution of problems. Indeed, the specific financing changes most vocally demanded are potentially very damaging to this approach.

## Requirements for future policy development

Potential changes in health financing systems must be assessed realistically to ensure that they will bring about an improvement in the current situation - resource shortages, resource inefficiencies and inequity. This discussion of existing problems of health systems and the problems of changing financing mechanisms is intended to help identify the actions necessary for the development of health financing systems within PHC.

The first requirement is to recognise that financing problems are part of national problems of resource constraints, and reflect existing national and health sector priorities. Isolated actions within the health sector are not enough; reallocation of resources from curative care to PHC will usually require the permission of the central government authorities. Additional support for PHC will only become continuously available when PHC is seen as a priority within the health sector and when the importance of health itself is recognised.

Secondly, raising the status of the health sector requires improved performance and, in particular, efficient use of available resources. There is clear evidence of inefficiency in many countries' health sectors; these undermine demands for more resources. Improved efficiency results from better management, appropriate training and incentives to manage. Such improvements will themselves help to address resource problems, by making more productive use of existing resources and by providing a basis for the successful implementation of new financing schemes. Additional revenues can make only a limited contribution if existing resources are not used efficiently.

### *Mobilising additional resources*

Given the range of possible financing mechanisms, it is important to first consider existing patterns of financing health activities and to establish a set of criteria with which to assess new options. Given the very different existing situations, what is possible will vary in each country. In Latin America more attention might be paid to containing cost inflation within health insurance systems than to introducing new systems; in some Asian countries the introduction of insurance schemes of a formal (e.g. in Korea) or informal (e.g. in Thailand) nature has been shown to be possible; in

Africa the demand for user fees and expanding community financing schemes is greatest.

However, the same general criteria can be applied everywhere to ensure that all of the potential effects of new systems are considered, and to ensure their compatibility with the PHC approach. WHO suggests seven criteria: equity, adequacy, reliability, impact on supply, impact on demand, intersectoral linkages and administrative feasibility. The Zairean financing approach outlined in the example above suggests alternative points. A central concern is that resource mobilisation efforts seek to reduce, rather than accentuate, inequity and thus are in line with the thrust of PHC.

Consideration should also be given to the role of the community in the process of system development. Are changes to be imposed from the top or generated from the bottom? Both approaches have problems, as the discussion of the Zairean experience and World Bank proposals indicates, but which is most likely to survive? In either approach it is essential to develop an effective, feasible and inexpensive exemption mechanism within fee systems. Without such a mechanism, equity will be undermined.

*Defining the equity goal of health systems*

More broadly, attention must be given to the development of a practical definition of the equity goal of health systems. How is equity pursued in a situation where resources are limited? The Zairean experience suggests one approach is to establish a minimum package of health care (a combination of preventive, basic curative and basic referral services) that must be provided in all regions of a country, and that will be financed by a fixed combination of government and community funds. Richer communities would be allowed to develop services above the minimum level if funds are available.

In such a strategy, equity is defined as equal provision of a minimum package of services. Is this adequate? Within communities an exemption mechanism could protect equity, but, beyond the minimum package of care, inequities between regions would be allowed. Is this acceptable? This strategy requires considerable decentralisation of decision making. Is this feasible? The government must continue to provide financial input to health services. Is this likely? Many questions are obviously raised by this approach, and hard decisions are required to develop strategies of 'financing with (some degree of) equity'.

*The importance of information*

A major weakness in the current health financing debates is the lack of relevant information. We do not know about the functioning of financing systems, about traditional financing practices, about the impact of newly introduced schemes. It is particularly important that all new schemes be monitored over a considerable length of time (at least five years) to learn their lessons and safeguard countries against problems. All this information must be gathered together and made accessible to a variety of audiences: the community, health programme managers and policy makers. Only this will allow the development of appropriate financing policies and ensure that health financing is not seen as the preserve of economists, but an area where all health workers can contribute to better understanding of ways to make effective improvements.

## References

Abel-Smit, B., 'The world economic crisis. Part 1: repercussions'. *Health Policy and Planning*, vol. 1, no. 3 (1986), pp. 202-213.

Attanayake, N. and U.H.S. De Silva, 'Economic analysis of health sector resource flows in Gampaha district of Sri Lanka' (unpublished).

Gilson, L., 'Government Health Care Charges: is Equity being Abandoned?' *EPC Publication no. 15* (1988). See especially Appendices I and II.

Janovsky, K. and A. Cassels, 'Strengthening district health systems based on Primary Health Care: report to the Division of Strengthening Health Services, WHO, Geneva, on a visit to the Ministry of Health, Ghana' (unpublished).

Janowitz, B. et al., 'Caesarian section in Brazil'. *Social Science and Medicine*, vol. 16, no. 1 (1982), pp. 19-25.

Musgrove, P., 'Measurement of equity in health'. *World Health Statistics Quarterly*, vol. 39, no. 4 (1986), pp. 325-335.

Ward, P., 'Reproduction of social inequality: access to health services in Mexico City'. *Health Policy and Planning*, vol. 2, no. 1 (1987), pp. 33-57.

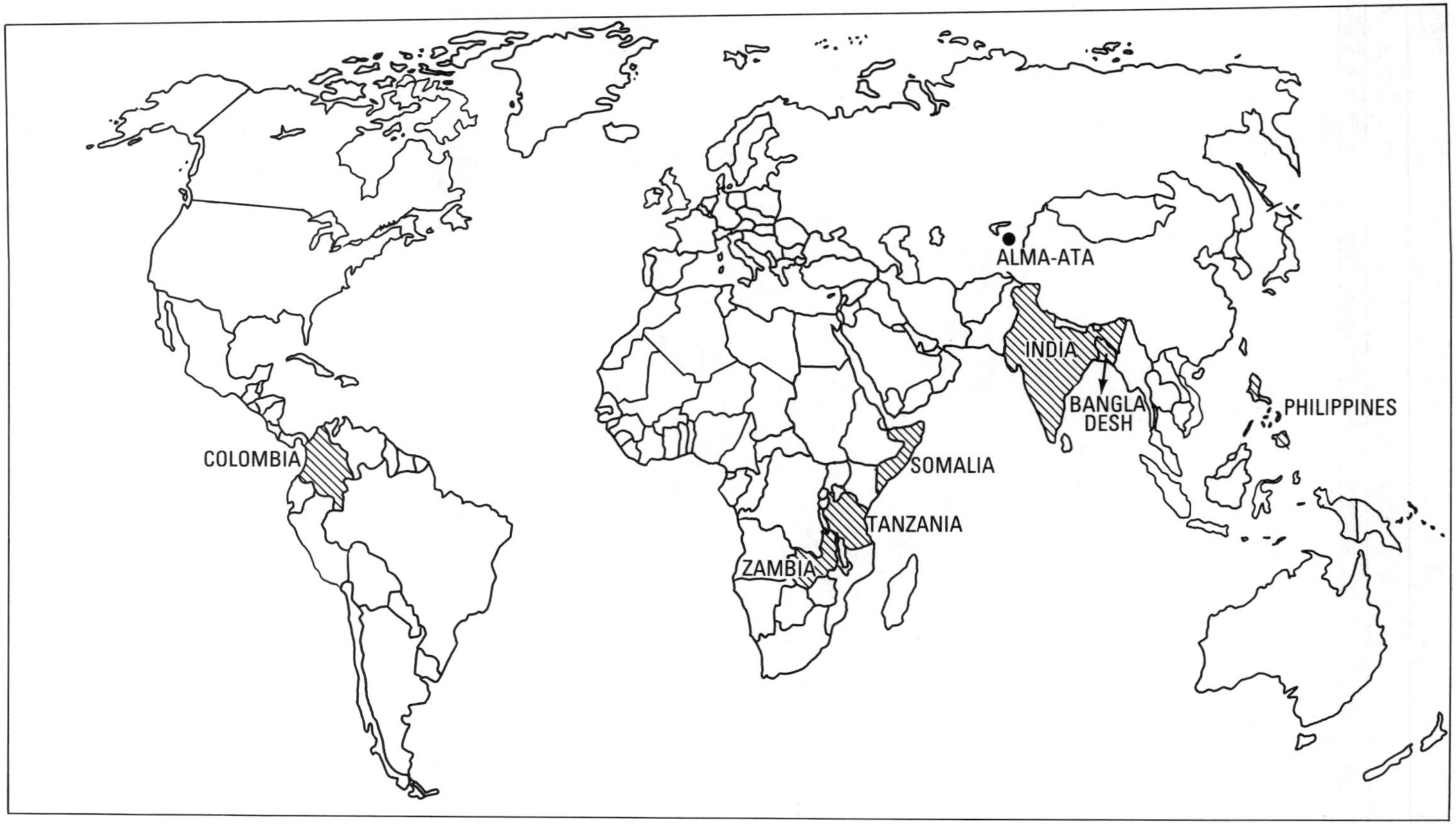


Shading denotes countries covered by case studies

Chapter 6

# Primary health care in northwest Somalia

*Chris Bentley*

Introducing primary health care usually involves a reorientation of conventional health services. Where an infrastructure is present, there is often a curative bias; the challenge is to incorporate effective preventive measures and improve knowledge of health and disease. But what of those areas where there is no effective health care infrastructure in the first place? In such cases community based programmes, rather than being extensions, become the service.

The primary health care project of the Ministry of Health in the Northwest of Somalia, assisted by UNICEF and initially also by Save the Children Fund (UK), found itself in such a situation. With conventional health services in a state of almost complete collapse except in the regional capital, the health needs of the rural population had to be addressed from scratch. Development of the project was made possible only by maintaining a very flexible approach, and by learning through doing. This paper is an attempt to identify some of the most important lessons learned along the way. Most are very practical points, which do not often feature in the extensive and ever growing PHC literature.

The project started in 1982; by 1986 it had reached a stage where progress appeared sufficient to warrant a formal review, which is also reported here.

## Somalia

Somalia is harsh territory situated in the Horn of Africa. It is sparsely populated: 5.5 million people occupy 640,000 square kilometres. However, some 900,000 refugees have arrived in recent years from Ethiopia. The Somali people are a homogeneous ethnic group with one religion (Islam) and language (Somali). About one half of the population is nomadic or semi-nomadic, depending for a livelihood on raising camels, sheep, goats and cattle. Twelve per cent of the population live in the capital, Mogadiscio. Much of the land is semi-arid scrub, and only a small percentage is accessible by vehicle. There is no railway, and telecommunications are not yet well developed.

The Somali Democratic Republic was established in 1960 as a result of the re-unification of the former British Somaliland Protectorate in the north and the Italian colony of Somaliland in the south. The present government took power in October 1969.

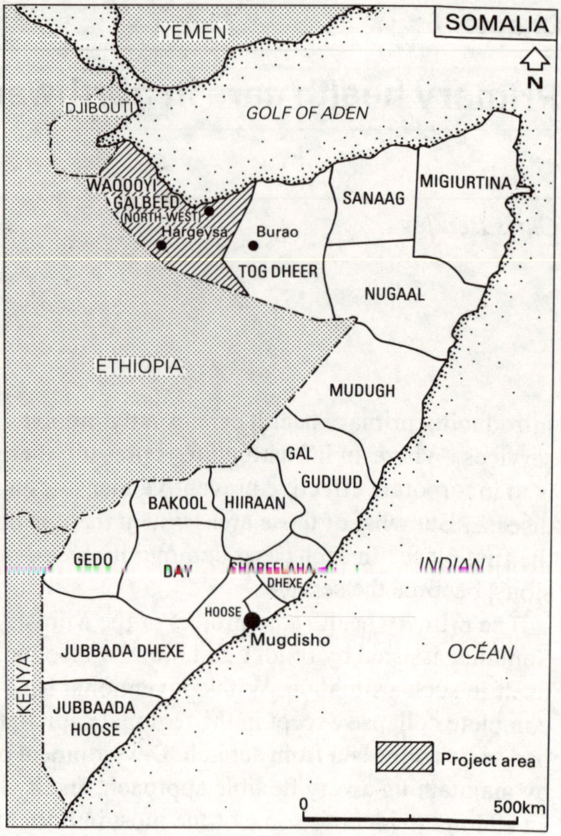


The country is divided, for administrative purposes, into 18 regions, which in turn comprise 85 districts.

Designated a least developed country by the United Nations, Somalia is one of the world's poorest nations, with a per capita income of approximately US$ 280. An adjustment programme was initiated in 1981, but despite three standby loans from the International Monetary Fund there has been little real economic growth. As a result, resources for social change in Somalia remain exceedingly limited. The social service sectors were thrown into disarray by the Ethiopian War of the late 1970s and the ensuing famine. Thus despite the successful campaign of the mid 1970s, literacy has again slumped to only 7% overall - probably the lowest in the world.

Health indicators also show a depressing picture. The crude death rate is 23 per 1,000. Child mortality is seventh highest in the world, at 257/1,000 live births; infant mortality is 152/1,000 live births. Maternal mortality is the third highest in the world, 1,100 per 100,000 live births.

The National Health Plan (1980-1985) recognised that 85-90% of the rural and nomadic population were out of reach of the national health services. Accordingly, the Ministry of Health began a reorientation to the primary health care approach. Donor support was sought for the development of regional programmes. UNICEF signed an

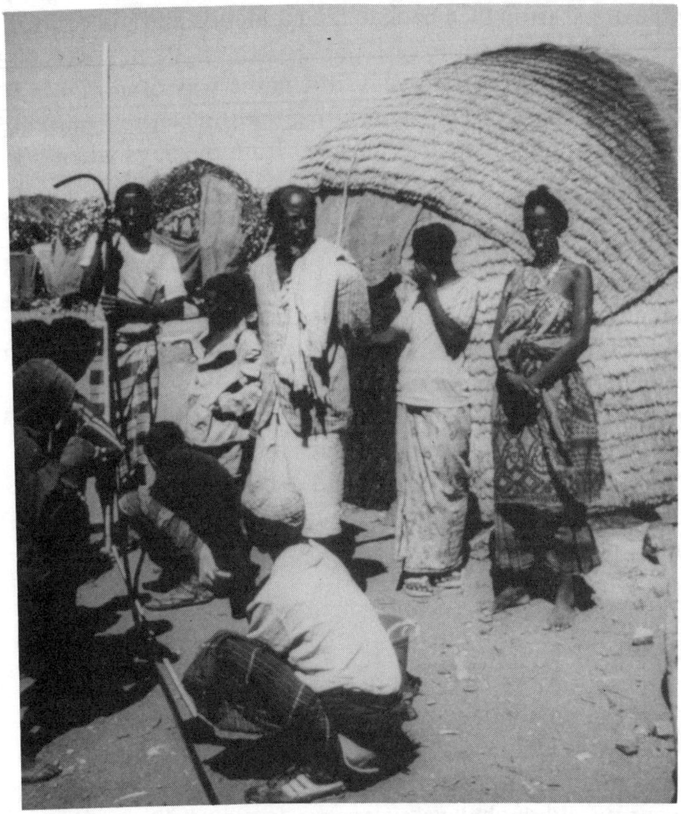

*Discussing the layout of the living environment in the Tuulo*

agreement with the government to provide financial and technical assistance to the Northwest region in September 1982. At the time of writing there were donor supported programmes in eleven of the 18 regions.

*The project area*

The Northwest of Somalia (six districts), formed the project area, some 44,000 square kilometres of semi-arid land. The estimated population is around 650,000, in an area with great diversity of topography, climate and population distribution.

Because of the semi-arid character of the land, the people's lifestyle is dictated to a large extent by the availability of water. Water is found principally in association with dry river beds (*togs*), or collected in man-made basins (*ballis* and *berkbads*). On the coast, water is found just below the surface, but tends to be brackish.

Largely because of these problems, only 2% of total land surface in the region is cultivated. Otherwise, land is cropped in the only efficient way: nomadic pastoralism involving sheep, goats and camels. The family economy is therefore most often based on pastoralism, but generally part of the family remains at a home base during wet seasons to grow sorghum and maize. This is primarily rain-fed cultivation, there being little irrigation. Thus there is a 'tidal' movement of the population down to the coast, where there is rainfall, during the dry season: then back to the highlands and plateau for the rainy season.

Although livestock is the region's main export, there is little in the way of a cash economy among nomads. The large villages that exist are either trading centres, market gardening areas supporting the towns, or marketplaces left over from the days when *qat* (a stimulant) was the major cash crop.

At sub-district level, the land is administratively divided into '*beels*', and within these into the smallest administrative units, '*tuulos*'. Each *tuulo* has a committee with an elected leader, and provides a representative for the *beel* committee. This structure arose out of the previous tribal organisation and now officially replaces it.

Within the *tuulos* there is considerable division of labour. Men are responsible for camel herding, most of the agricultural work and almost all political and administrative dealings. Women and older children look after small stock such as the sheep, goats and chickens; collect wood and water; cook and prepare food; and of course look after the young children. In commercial centres women generally run markets and shops. Tea shops, however, are a purely male domain.

## Programme strategy and process

Health services in the region were extremely run down in 1982. With services already stretched, the refugee influx that settled in nine camps with almost half a million people, many in extremis, was a further drain. Establishing a health care system for refugees drained personnel resources, although the assistance programme did produce an influx of medical supplies, drugs and equipment.

The basis of the regional health care infrastructure was a regional hospital, which was well staffed and moderately well supplied with government and donor resources. Beyond this was supposed to be a hospital and maternal and child health centre in each district capital, and a series of dispensaries. Of these six hospitals two were non-functional; the others were run-down, poorly staffed, un-supplied and hardly used. Maternal and child health centres were receiving no regular supplies other than supplementary rations. Only three of 21 registered dispensaries were in any way functional.

Programme strategy was shaped primarily by the fact that very little health service existed outside district capitals. This was due mainly to lack of staff and reluctance of trained staff to become residents in isolated rural areas. There were three major consequences:

- it was necessary to use a mobile district team to carry out training, supervision and support of village level staff;
- there were to be no peripheral referral points: the bulk of curative work was to be carried out by community level staff. This included sophisticated treatments such as antibiotics, and procedures such as suturing and management of major trauma;

• dependence on (trainee) district nurse teams for all forms of community support had an additional consequence: only a few community programmes could be started initially; expansion could only occur as the capacity of teams increased.

*Management*

Rather than being tightly planned and implemented, the project evolved. The decision was made to maintain a flexible approach, so that plans could be constantly modified on the basis of new information and experience.

The basis of the management process was a meeting each six months of regional team staff. At each meeting performance was reviewed and plans established for the next six months. Reviews and plans of action were structured around a series of twelve objectives, each with sub-objectives. This structure ensured that all key areas of the programme, including budgeting and logistic details, were both planned for and reviewed. This was a vital learning process for a staff untrained in management process. A six month planning cycle was the most it was practical for national staff to handle.

Within each six month period, management depended on a monthly cycle of preparation and review of workplans. Tactics were decided by the regional team, but details were worked out by district teams. The main step towards this arrangement came with the decision to 'block' a period at the end of each month, when district teams would spend three to four days in the regional capital. The main tasks to be undertaken were:

• workplans: debriefing teams on previous month's workplan, planning of next month's workplan;
• collection of health information: handing in collected village data on mortality, morbidity, births, rainfall, market prices, vaccination figures and campaign reports;
• village-by-village review: debriefings for each village visited, problems analysed and solutions planned, allowing teams to develop some continuity of approach;
• education/training: debriefings provided an opportunity to teach, and a journal club was used to introduce new materials;
• vehicle control and maintenance: servicing of team cars, log book check, fuel provision;
• provision of essential drugs and vaccines;
• payment of salaries and incentives;
• opportunity for teams to meet and compare notes.

One of the most important results of this system was the early involvement of all middle level staff in 'management'.

*Orientation and selection at community level*

The number of communities to be involved initially was limited by the supervisory capacity of the mobile teams. The larger, more centralised communities, usually the *beel* centres, were chosen first. This allowed maximum coverage early, and provided a base for expansion into surrounding smaller *tuulos*.

Orientation took place in a series of visits by regional and district team members to each selected village. Meetings were held with the village committee and the community as a whole. Representatives of committees from each batch of new villages were then invited to a joint orientation day. Each such day ended with presentation of suggested criteria for selecting candidates for community health worker training. After the meeting communities were invited to appoint a health subcommittee of the village committee. The first task of this group was to oversee the selection of health workers. Suggested criteria included:

- permanent residency in the *tuulo*, preferably with family;
- history of previous community service if possible;
- age between 20 and 45 years;
- not a close relative of any member of the central or health committee;
- literacy.

Final selection of candidates, who were generally male, was approved after an interview by the district PHC team. There were rejections, but in general selections seemed appropriate.

*Training*

*Regional and district teams.* This was one of the first PHC projects in the country; Ministry of Health staff in the region had very little knowledge or experience of the PHC approach, except for some who had worked in the refugee health programme. This excellent programme had developed a national body, the Refugee Health Unit, which utilised a primary health care approach and had established a methodology, sets of guidelines, and management, information and logistic systems for the network of camps throughout the country. Some of the very good staff identified by this programme were used to form a core group for national PHC programmes. They contributed a well founded PHC approach and a basis for disease management guidelines. Further in-service training was provided for this group by assigning them as counterparts to expatriate technical staff.

All district team staff received a four month training course at a nearby post-basic school, including elements of public health nursing, sanitation, midwifery and laboratory work. Within the regional programme, training was initially very much in-service based, plus a series of quarterly one to two week training workshops.

*Community health workers.* Design of the first training course for community health workers (CHWs) was of vital importance for the success of the community based programme. The following points were considered:

- teaching method: the majority of candidates were farmers, herdsmen or tea shop boys. Very few had any formal education other than the massive nationwide literacy campaign initiated in 1976. Most teaching therefore centred on discussion groups and practical work;
- course duration: for a significant proportion of students, the course was their first time away from 'home', and in the big town. A course that was too long might be counterproductive;
- course content: candidates were unlikely to be able to absorb too much at the first attempt, since everything would be totally new. The orientation to PHC, the CHW role

and the causation of disease alone would be very demanding, before any 'clinical' topics had even been introduced.

The final design divided the training as follows:
- first course, duration three weeks:
  week 1: orientation;
  week 2: 'clinical' topics;
  week 3: practical application of new knowledge;
- in-service work, four to six months:
- second course, duration four weeks:
  week 1: refresher course and problem solving;
  week 2-3: new clinical topics;
  week 4: practical application of new knowledge;
- refresher course, one week every six months.

The orientation week addressed PHC concepts, CHW role, structure of the community, germ theory of disease and the wider definition of health. Here maximum use was made of contact with other health workers and institutions. Refugee camps were of particular value: the PHC approach was being successfully used, and students could see implementation by grassroots workers with cultural backgrounds similar to their own.

In the first course, clinical content was restricted to three to four subjects, selected on the basis of priority need expressed by communities. The commonest topics were anaemia, malaria, diarrhoea/dehydration and vaccination. This combination was felt to contain a good balance of education, prevention and simple treatments. It was accepted that some difficulties would be experienced when, being unable to treat common complaints such as coughs, eye disease and wounds, CHWs failed to meet the high expectations of their communities. It was preferable, however, not to overload them at first. Respiratory infections, eye and skin diseases and first aid were taught in the longer second course, when CHWs were intent on absorbing as much knowledge as possible to meet community expectations. Some basics of nutrition and personal, domestic and environmental hygiene were taught in both courses.

The final week of the first course attempted to prepare students for the reality of the job, examining what their new theoretical knowledge was to mean in practice. Field visits, secondment to a refugee camp, a maternal and child health clinic, a hospital ward, and participation in vaccination sessions served to 'throw them in the deep end' while help was still at hand. Role playing was a very valuable tool. Drama, poetry and song are basic to Somali culture. Role playing thus comes naturally and is enjoyed by all. Such sessions as the 'home visit', the 'health committee meeting' and 'teaching the mother to prepare oral rehydration salts' allowed an informed and detailed examination of potential problems in a way that was easy and memorable.

Experience suggested visual aids would be of limited use. In a rural society of few artifacts and a strong oral tradition, slides and pictures had novelty value, but their information was not easily retained. Initially, the written word was also not well absorbed (from the blackboard or printed handouts). However, the course notes, whether handwritten by students or on duplicated sheets were invaluable in the long term. In the months following the course, the students were found to have read and re-read their materials. This was excellent for retention of facts such as symptom complexes and drug dosages.

Much learning was done 'out of hours'. The group of students spent most of this time together in the dormitory and at meals, and never seemed to stop discussing the new information and ideas. This applied to practical techniques as well. For example, many found it difficult to read a thermometer at first. However, when two or three had mastered it, all students were given thermometers. Within 48 hours all were proficient. On the whole, students were very bright and learned easily. Many seemed hungry for knowledge and constantly asked intelligent questions.

The major part of the teaching has been carried out by a few key individuals. Initially, the intention was to ensure that district teams would do most of the teaching. However, many of these sessions were so poorly delivered that re-runs were required. Eventually, the natural teachers were selected and used exclusively, with other members helping out in practical ways.

*Health committees.* Health committee members were vital in their own right, particularly for promotional and educational parts of the programme. Members were all elders and were looked to for wisdom and advice. CHWs, who were generally much younger and less well respected, were accepted for their specialist curative knowledge, but suggestions on changing behaviour or carrying out preventive activities such as well or latrine digging needed the backing of those older and wiser. Therefore a series of training sessions were held specifically for health committee members. These courses tended to follow on from the CHW six-month refresher courses. Some time overlap was allowed, to allow for joint sessions. This also provided opportunities for CHWs to put on a drama for a wider audience, which was very beneficial.

*Supplies and logistics*

An essential drugs list, based on that of the Refugee Health Unit, was standardised at regional level and subsequently adopted, with a few modifications, for the National Programme. This list formed the basis for an essential drugs programme. Drugs and supplies were imported through UNIPAC, and received into a central store in the regional capital. Here district allocations were packed on a two monthly cycle, and collected by the district teams during their management meetings. District teams were then responsible for delivering drugs directly to communities. District level stores were discouraged; teams visited all their communities over a three day period at the beginning of the cycle. Allocations were not fixed, and a dynamic system of requests, checks and returns was established. Supervision was the basis for the success of the system.

A similar system was also established to provide a cold chain for vaccines. Here supplies came from the National Central Cold Chain in the capital and district level cold chain units were established. District teams were responsible for vaccination programmes, carrying six-day cold boxes on their community visits; they relied on health committee and CHW work to prepare communities in advance.

The dependence of all support work on the vehicle fleet was recognised by the establishment of the Transport and Equipment Maintenance Operation Workshop. This facility operated a system of regular preventive maintenance and repair for trucks and land rovers/land cruisers. There was also a limited training programme for driver/ mechanics. Fuel was imported especially for the programme and stored in regional and district level stations.

*Development of approach*

The planning and implementation process of the first four years can be seen in two distinct phases. The first two years were spent working out ground rules, training service staff and setting up systems and infrastructures. This entire phase was required to establish the credibility of the programme with the communities served.

In phase two, this functional infrastructure was used to address targets related to child and maternal survival objectives. This phase involved a major reorientation of approach, introducing the concept of coverage. Previously, the programme had been rural, limited to a small number of villages. Now, its aims were wider: it looked toward rapid rural expansion and development of an urban dimension.

The rapid expansion programme in phase two required a rationalisation of approach. The greater workload limited the individual tailoring possible for community programmes. Some compromise was made possible, however, by the recognition of three main types of communities:

• Type A: a settled village where the majority of the population resides in the centre. Trading is the main source of income, but there is a settled agricultural base. Most *beel* centres are of this type.

• Type B: has a smaller centre; the majority of the population live in satellites around the centre. Agriculture is the basis of the economy, with some cattle, but all families also have a nomadic element.

• Type C: a pastoralist community, diffuse and mobile. The centre consists of tea shops and a meeting hut. There is little agriculture. During the predominant season, the community tends to move within the *tuulo*, but they usually migrate seasonally or as rainfall and grazing dictate.

Classification of villages into these types immediately allowed a diversification in the strategies used by district teams. In type A villages a 'clinic' type service was found to be developing. CHWs were tending to sit in their health posts, where they offered treatment but little education and few preventive initiatives. To attempt to reverse this trend, a system of family registration was developed, in which the CHW was expected to visit each family each month to update forms, including:

• vaccination status of under-fives;

• registration of new pregnancies and record of iron and chloroquine prophylaxis;

• recording of sanitation arrangements and water source, followed by monthly record of diarrhoea episodes.

This has been effective in refocusing CHW work toward priority issues.

In type B villages, CHWs were making frequent rounds of the satellites. There were limitations, however, in contacts with women. Diarrhoea episodes were a particular problem. When children had diarrhoea, frequently it was the husband who came to the centre to collect medicine. Oral rehydration salts were provided, but apparently little information transfer was occurring from husband to wife. The CHW had no direct contact with the mother so as to be able to advise and teach. In a new strategy, each satellite elected a woman helper or '*gargarooyin*'. This person became the key informant for the CHW in that satellite. She was trained in the use of oral rehydration therapy and preparation of oral rehydration salts (ORS), and in the importance and methods of prevention of anaemia in pregnancy. This woman, who was often also the traditional birth attendant (TBA), was supplied with ORS, iron and chloroquine by the CHW, from his stock.

In type C *tuulos*, the main priority need expressed has always been animal health. For these communities, a system is being developed for reimbursable procurement of veterinary drugs by health committees, and education of CHWs by the District Veterinarian in their use.

*Traditional birth attendants*

It has always been intended that training or upgrading of TBAs should be an integral part of the programme. After the initial wave of CHW training, a detailed survey of knowledge, attitudes and practice about delivery and the post-partum period was carried out. The survey was conducted in twelve villages, including some of each 'type' (A, B and C). Thirty mothers chosen randomly were interviewed in depth. Subsequently, each birth attendant mentioned by these mothers was interviewed, using a different questionnaire. The available referral facilities and their services were also reviewed. These investigations made apparent that a 'conventional' TBA programme would not be realistic. The main reasons were:

*Lack of referral facilities*. Conventional TBA programmes have relied for their main impact on detection of 'at risk' pregnancies, and referral to appropriately staffed and equipped facilities, such as maternal and child health centres and hospitals. In the project area little was to be gained by detecting those 'at risk', because of the poor access of the majority of the population to referral centres and the inadequate staffing, level of training and standard of facilities in referral centres.

*Restricted use of TBAs*. Traditionally, TBAs have no recognised function in the antenatal period. In the survey they were seen in all cases to be called and involved only for a 72 hour period around the time of delivery. Remuneration was by an 'in kind' payment, usually of food and drink related to the cultural 'rites' associated with a birth, e.g. slaughtering an animal. No TBAs were full time 'professionals'; all were otherwise fully occupied with domestic activity. Only the emergency of an actual delivery warranted time away from home.

*Lack of 'professional' TBAs in most areas.* The pattern of assistance for deliveries differed with the structure of the community:

• type A *tuulos*: one or two TBAS served most of the population in the concentrated centres. Some assisted up to twenty deliveries a month,

• type B *tuulos*: each of the 8-15 satellites had one or two TBAS, each seeing only one or two deliveries per month,

• type C *tuulos*: in these diffuse communities, each grandmother was a 'TBA', helping in perhaps five deliveries a year.

Thus only in the few type A villages would training one or two individuals possibly produce an impact on mortality and morbidity.

*Problems in educating existing TBAs.* The majority of TBAS were old, and all were illiterate. Less than 10% were prepared to travel away from the village for extra training, and none of these for periods longer than three days.

*Quality and quantity of midwives available for training.* Since no midwives had been trained in Somalia for a number of years, staffing levels were particularly low. The majority available were middle aged, with family commitments. They were thus unwilling to undertake the extensive and arduous travel commitment required for training and supervision.

These major difficulties meant considerable effort would be required to construct a viable programme, with small expected gains: the survey showed a very high standard of umbilical cord care, and good knowledge and health practices regarding delivery skills in the majority of TBAS. There was a very low incidence of neonatal tetanus. The major problem was post-partum haemorrhage, compounded by the high prevalence of anaemia and obstructed labour.

Although the intent is still to establish an educational programme for TBAS, this will concentrate initially on type A villages. Meanwhile, an attempt is being made to attack maternal/child death due to post-partum haemorrhage by utilising CHWS to deliver iron and chloroquine prophylaxis to pregnant women in an attempt to reduce anaemia, and by making ergometrine available to communities, again initially through CHWS.

## Evaluation

Four years after the inception of the programme, a variant of the WHO standard PHC review was carried out in Northwest Somalia. Selected *tuulos* were surveyed in four of the six districts. The 24 index communities were chosen randomly from a list of names by the external evaluators; where possible, these were matched with non-PHC controls (12 villages).

Evaluation teams were a mixture of district, regional and national level Somali staff, and external evaluators from agencies within and outside Somalia. The evaluation was used as a training exercise for national staff, as well as providing useful review data on the programme, as summarised below.

*Regional and district levels: personnel*

Quantitatively, the trained personnel available were found to be limited. However, external evaluators found regional team members to be a very capable, innovative and hardworking core group. The middle management level of district team and health unit staff was unfortunately a different story. There are four main reasons:

• inadequate basic training: the nursing course in the regional capital of Hargeisa was held in English, in which only a small proportion of students were proficient. Also, the course included only a very minor component on community health and preventive medicine;

• curative service bias: most staff came from curative services, and had no community health experience;

• inappropriate training: all staff were sent for four months to a post-basic school for orientation and re-training. Unfortunately, the course was totally inadequate. The curriculum, based on standard 'Western' public health nurse training, was not tailored to the Somali situation. There were no components on management, survey techniques or training methods. Facilities were inadequate. Re-orientation of graduates by regional PHC staff was required before the programme could start;

• poor staff motivation: the small National Health budget provides only a very inadequate salary. At the start of the programme a nurse earned only the equivalent of US$ 36 per month, which has now fallen to US$ 7 due to devaluations and inflation. Even with incentives and travel allowances provided by the programme, it is impossible to live on this income alone. In consequence, most staff leave civil service employment after a few years to establish themselves in the private sector. District teams thus tend to remain young and inexperienced due to turnover.

Several approaches have been tried to rectify the middle management gap, but with very limited success. Without major changes in training and conditions of employment, intensive supervision from above is required to achieve even a routine level of service. The lack of reliability, innovation and creativity at this important interface between the health service and the village based programmes is a major constraint.

In addition to the problem of staff quality, there has been consistent understaffing of district teams. In particular there have been insufficient sanitarians and midwives to bring all teams up to specifications. It is of course particularly difficult to obtain staff for the more remote districts where living conditions are harsh.

*Fieldwork*

As mentioned, supervision and support have been problem areas due to quality, quantity and poor motivation of district team staff. Much regional team effort was expended initially just ensuring regularity of visits. This had paid dividends, and the frequent contact and reliable provision of drugs and supplies has established community confidence in the programme. CHWs questioned during the review reported an average number of supervisory visits ranging from 0.9 to 1.3 per month, varying from district to district. This exceeded the target of once every six weeks.

Teams demonstrated enthusiasm for direct service activities, in particular vaccination sessions. Referral work has also held their interest. However, their capability in this regard has not been good and it has been difficult to develop a logical progression of diagnostic or treatment protocols based on initial contact of patient with CHW. This is largely due to poor basic nursing training, but also reflects an initial emphasis: since project management skills had not previously been taught, these were the focus of most early workshops and supervision. As a result, teams began to see their jobs in terms of drug delivery, completion of forms, checking on register books, and discussing CHW payment with health committees.

*Community leadership: tuulo committee*

All *tuulos* but one had a committee: usually there are five to eight members, all males, selected by District Commissioners. The Chairman is a member of the Party. Meetings are held twice a month in most cases.

The *tuulo* committee leaves health matters to the health committee if there is one. Otherwise, they incidentally discuss health matters, such as disease outbreaks, and report to the District.

*Tuulo health committee*

All 24 PHC villages had a health committee. In one village the committee was functioning badly, but in all others the committees appeared active, and met at least once monthly.

The average health committee has four to five members and included one woman. Most of male members are also members of the *tuulo* committee. The role of women in the health committee varies. In a few villages they were reportedly outspoken and were considered experts in mother and child health. In others the impression prevails that women are added to the committee only because the District/Regional team encourages this.

Committees have been gradually reshaped during the life of the programme; they are now far more representative of satellite areas and occupation groups. Establishing a working female presence on committees has always been an uphill battle, however. Partly this is due to male prejudice and a tradition that men do the 'public speaking'. Mainly, though, it is due to the heavy domestic workload. Women genuinely do not have the time, particularly when meetings would involve significant travel time to go to the centre.

As the health committees gradually took on a functioning role, the importance of the strong link with the village committee became apparent. Through this channel, the committee maintains access to the established local balance of tribal connections and modern party-based administration, which form the local communication and decision making machinery.

Meetings are as frequent as once a week. Major topics are discussion of individual problems, making a workplan for the CHW, discussion of disease prevention in the village and organisation of immunisation days. Health committees are also involved in collection of remuneration for CHWs; cleanliness campaigns; health education; organising transport for very sick persons; reporting cases from their village sectors to the CHW and monitoring the work of the CHW.

*CHW selection and personal characteristics*
In the 24 PHC villages, a total of 30 CHWs were interviewed as part of the review. All were male, half were married. The mean age is 29 years, with a range of 18 to 45 years (see Table 1). Fourteen CHWs had been selected by the community, six by the village health committee or village committee, two by the health committee and community together, and two by community leaders.

Table 1. Age distribution of CHWs (in years)

| Age | Number |
|---|---|
| <20 | 1 |
| 20-24 | 5 |
| 25-29 | 10 |
| 30-34 | 8 |
| 35-39 | 2 |
| 40+ | 2 |
| unknown | 2 |

The infrequency with which female candidates had been appointed was a disappointment. There were several reasons: it was very difficult to find literate women, or women who could be spared from work within the family; and the work, involving much walking and visiting of households in isolated settings, was not culturally acceptable for women. This was a very real problem for those few female CHWs who were appointed.

*Educational background and level of knowledge*
Schooling levels are generally low (Table 2); the majority learned to read and write during the 1976 literacy campaign, but had no other formal education.

Table 2. Source of schooling

| Schooling | Number |
|---|---|
| elementary school | 8 |
| literacy campaign | 12 |
| Qu'ran school | 2 |
| other | 8 |

The level of knowledge of the CHWs was assessed, using questions on signs of dehydration, immunisation schedules and pneumonia symptoms and treatment. A nine point scale was used, with five indicating an adequate level. The level of knowledge was found to be very high. Most CHWs scored eight points. CHWs generally expressed satisfaction with their training. Most had had a refresher course within the previous six month period.

*Workload*

CHWs usually work five to seven days per week, including some night work. The average number of hours worked per day was six; the number of hours varied from four to more than eight. Although it is difficult to obtain an accurate estimate (no records of home visits are kept), the number of household visits is very high. Many CHWs make two to four complete rounds of their villages each month, and the mean number of household visits is often over 100. A question about the number of people or households served elicited a broad range of responses. Two CHWs claimed to serve more than 7,000 people; seven said fewer than 1,000. Their estimates are probably not very accurate, and vary by type of village. Some villages have many remote satellites that cannot be served routinely by CHWs.

Main activities, in order of importance, are: treatment of common illnesses, care of children and mothers, sanitation activities, and health education talks. Oral rehydration therapy and control of diarrhoeal diseases (which, if combined, would be number one), and birth and death registration come next.

All CHWs but three kept records. This included a treatment book, rainfall records, family forms and a register of pregnant women (iron and chloroquine prophylaxis). The average standard of record keeping was high, but utilisation for planning, analysis, etc. was limited.

*Community support*

The population to be reached in each *tuulo* showed a variety of socio-cultural, economic and political features. Therefore it was decided that the initial choice of a payment mechanism was to be made by each community, without project interference. The only stipulation was that a fee-for-service system would not be acceptable. Such a system would discourage promotion of preventive services, and might defeat the aim of reaching the poorest of the poor, for whom any price might be too high.

During the first two to three years of the programme, much time and effort was expended in following up on community commitment to CHW payment. Without pressure from project staff, there was almost universal failure to meet promises for regular remuneration. This was the main and often sole topic on the agenda for health committee meetings with district teams. Fortunately, concern that CHWs would lose heart and stop working was not borne out in practice. Of 85 trained, only 10 had dropped out by the end of 1985. The reasons given were:

- all three female CHWs left, one to re-marry, one because her family did not accept the travel involved and one to obtain higher education in the Middle East;
- one male CHW was dismissed by a council of other CHWs because he had been involved in smuggling activities;
- two good candidates, brought to public attention by their health activities, were hired away by local businessmen;
- one left to take over family businesses from retiring parents;
- one, apparently a deserter from the army, left the country to escape charges;

• two from one *tuulo* left very early in the programme when the community decided it did not need extra services, since there was a large refugee camp immediately adjacent, with a very good health system.

Most of these workers have been replaced by training new candidates at the request of the committees concerned.

Why does work continue? There are many contributing factors:

• it is very rare for *no* payment to be given. Presents of cigarettes, sugar, grain, etc. are often given periodically by the elders. In many cases, bachelor CHWs are provided with accommodation, rent free. Also, while making home visits to sick people there will often be some form of payment in kind, such as a meal, container of milk, or meat if available (as it often is when there is a sick family member);

• even a CHW working hard at his job usually owns a farm and herd, which his family looks after. At harvest season, or when herds have to be moved, he will return to help. Thus, anything derived from health activities is extra income;

• rewards such as increased standing in the community and, in a community deprived of learning opportunities, the intellectual satisfaction of new learning, are very important. These can even be sufficient alone, particularly in times of drought/famine when everybody understands that little is left over from family budgets.

An analysis in November 1985, during which in-depth interviews were conducted with CHWs and health committee members from all villages, showed that the payment situation was improving. House-to-house collection proved difficult and time consuming in many villages; a variety of more viable alternatives were found:

• water tax on the village hand-pump (installed with UNICEF assistance). 1 Somali shilling (SSh) per household and 5 SSh per tea shop per day provides a fund to pay a CHW salary as well as pump spares, lubricants and watchmen;

• shop and tea shop cash collection. The larger villages found that a levy collected in tea shops reduced footwork, provided good public relations for the shops, and was satisfying because travellers were indirectly supporting community health;

• insurance-type collection. Payment of a small fee assured regular visits by the CHW. Poorer families were added to the list without payment, at the discretion of the health committee;

• once yearly livestock collection. In many villages, payment in kind is more practical. A number of nomadic communities were paying with livestock once herds had survived the dry season;

• once yearly grain collection. Agricultural communities paid after harvest;

• waived fee for water rights, this applied to CHW's family herds;

• payment by a wealthy local landowner. This became less common after the main cash crop, *qat*, was banned.

The results of this analysis and the various payment methodologies became the basis for a health committee workshop in early 1986. Many villages then adopted one of the new payment methods, and the proportion providing reliable support dramatically improved and was maintained throughout the year.

During the review, all of the CHWs interviewed indicated receipt of payments, mostly on a monthly basis, but sometimes very irregularly. Eighteen of these CHWs were able to state a specific amount received each month. The lowest was SSh 500, the highest SSh 2,000.

*Household impact: CHW utilisation.* As shown in Table 3, interviews at household level during the review showed that in the PHC *tuulos*, 89% knew the CHW and 74% were visited by the CHW during the previous two months. In households with someone ill, 75% went to the CHW in the PHC *tuulos* and 19% in the non-PHC villages. Traditional healers were visited in slightly over 10% of all cases.

Table 3. CHW utilisation in *tuulos*

| | | PHC + | PHC - |
|---|---|---|---|
| CHW known: | yes | 89% | |
| | no | 11% | |
| Visited in last months: | yes | 74% | |
| | no | 26% | |
| Where did you go the last time any member of the family was ill? | | | |
| • government facility | | 7% | 25% |
| • traditional healer | | 10% | 16% |
| • CHW | | 75% | 19% |
| • pharmacy | | 1% | 11% |
| • other | | 4% | 27% |

It is interesting to note that even in non-PHC villages, only 16% of sick people visited traditional healers first, even though visits to government facilities, pharmacies and 'other' would require long, difficult travel. It would seem that 'modern' medicine is preferred to traditional. Exceptions to this, in the experience of project staff, are mental illness and fractures, treated by *sheiks* and bone-setters respectively.

Thus it appears that the work of the CHW is well accepted; the use of his services confirms the previous need. That 19% of sick people in non-PHC *tuulos* also sought out a CHW similarly confirms their acceptability.

*Effect on disease and management.* The review addressed the effect of the programme on disease management via changes in management of diarrhoeal episodes. This had been identified as the major health problem during baseline survey work.

Treatment patterns for diarrhoea in under-fives are shown in Table 4. ORS are used by 58% of mothers in PHC villages; an additional 20% use homemade fluids. Drugs and other treatments are rarely used. In control villages, fluids were given by half of the mothers, but ORS are also given by 15%. This is most likely a spillover from CHW activities in neighbouring PHC villages (or nomads who carried knowledge with them). Another significant difference between PHC and non-PHC villages is in the percentage who did nothing when their child had diarrhoea: 14% in PHC villages, versus 28% in non-PHC villages.

Table 4. Diarrhoea treatment patterns

| | PHC + | | PHC - | |
|---|---|---|---|---|
| | No. | % | No. | % |
| ORS | 53 | ( 57.6 ) | 7 | ( 14.9 ) |
| home fluids | 18 | ( 19.6 ) | 23 | ( 48.9 ) |
| drugs and other | 8 | ( 8.7 ) | 4 | ( 8.5 ) |
| nil | 13 | ( 14.1 ) | 13 | ( 27.7 ) |
| Total | 92 | (100.0 ) | 47 | (100.0 ) |

Of women in PHC villages, 66% mentioned at least one way of preventing diarrhoea, most commonly keeping food clean. In villages without PHC, only 37% could specify a way to prevent diarrhoea.

*Disease prevention.* Despite improved knowledge in PHC villages about causation and ways to prevent diarrhoea, diarrhoea incidence in the two weeks before the survey was 15.7% in PHC villages and 14.5% in other villages. There were an average of four episodes of diarrhoea per child per year. The age pattern showed the expected variation, with peak incidence at 6-11 and 12-23 months, corresponding with the weaning period. It is clear there is no significant difference in diarrhoea incidence in these two groups.

The lack of change reflects missing inputs related to water source and sanitation hardware. These aspects of the planned integrated approach have been neglected, as water and sanitation projects have not kept up with the advances of the health programme.

## Conclusion

Over a four year period, it has been possible to establish a functioning and effective health service infrastructure in an area where there was effectively none before. There are still many problems, and in particular there is considerable dependence on outside inputs - particularly drugs, fuel and transport. However, the system, which is largely managed by national staff, has won the support of constituent communities, who now contribute to improving their own health status.

It has proved possible to train grassroots level workers with no previous education, only basic literacy, and no previous health background to carry out even fairly sophisticated curative work with little supervision, and to develop a high level of knowledge.

Despite initial problems, communities have been persuaded to take some responsibility for their own health, and to voluntarily commit their own resources. The main factors in this process were an appropriate level of service, tailored to perceived needs; and building up credibility for the PHC system by concentrating on establishing a regular and reliable support system. Once immediate curative needs had been met, communities were very interested in acquiring new knowledge to help improve their own health.

The most difficult part of the programme was the attempt to develop a middle management structure. In general, the personnel milieu in the health service is counterproductive. Very low level incentives, poor and inappropriate training and uncertain career development opportunities all contribute to low morale and high turnover. Programme successes have largely been based on identifying high potential individuals at all levels, who have been developed by means of intensive counterparting with expatriate staff. This has yielded good results, but produced a very vulnerable structure. There is little in depth strength.

For the future, it is vital that systems be designed to produce cadres of appropriately trained staff, particularly with developed management and teaching skills. This must be addressed at national, not programme level.

## Postscript

Tragically, during 1988, a destructive civil war of a mainly tribal nature broke out in Somalia, starting in the Northwest. The population of the regional capital, Hargeisa, was reduced from 250,000 to a reported 5,000 in early 1989, as survivors of the fighting and the air strikes fled. All forms of official social service completely broke down, including, of course, the health services. Vehicles were taken for military use and drugs and medical equipment commandeered. Staff and health workers were either conscripted to work in the military hospitals, fled to join the 'rebels', or crossed as refugees into Ethiopia. Many PHC staff and CHWs have been encountered by workers for Save the Children Fund in the camps in the Ogaden, where they are using their training to good effect, helping with medical services. All expatriates have been forced to evacuate.

This thoroughly depressing state of affairs, however, does not signal the end of PHC in the Northwest. Firstly, the lessons of the 'experiment' have been learnt and built upon. Other programmes inside and, hopefully, outside Somalia have benefited from the project experience. Secondly, the communities involved have seen that a community based approach is more effective than conventional services, and they have experienced the benefits of participation and of taking more responsibility for their own health. When, in due course, order returns, hopefully people will aspire to a restoration of their primary care programme. Finally, a body of young, intelligent and enterprising workers have developed knowledge and experience of an approach that has worked in Somalia, and that hopefully they can develop there once again.

Chapter 7

# Experiences from the Maasai Health Services Project in Tanzania

*E.M. Nangawe*

Twenty-seven years ago Tanzania became independent. Its population, which was then around 8 million people, has since trebled. This paper reviews the development trends of the past 10 years, which can largely be viewed as a period of economic depression and regression in the country. The war with Uganda's Idi Amin, the subsequent drought, and general economic recession in the world have occasioned almost insurmountable difficulties for the national economy. The national currency devalued to one fifth of its value (relative to the US dollar) at the beginning of the decade.

With such a severe depression it is not surprising that health has received relatively less and less of the national budget in recent years: in 1972/73 the allocation was 8.9% of the national budget; comparable figures for 1980s are between 5.6 and 5.2% (Mahalu et al., 1986).

## Tanzania's health care system

There are three main levels in the government health care system: district hospitals, regional hospitals and consultant hospitals. Auxiliary services are provided two levels below the district hospital: the rural or urban health centre and the dispensary.
An attempt to extend wider coverage of services to communities has been made by training village health workers. Of late this has received increasing emphasis. Among NGOs, community based health care has become the focus of attention, rather than a mere extension of the health care tiers.

Referrals go from dispensary to rural health centre to district and regional hospitals; for geographic convenience, regional hospitals may receive cases from nearby health centres (usually urban based). Consultant hospitals get referral cases from regional hospitals and specialised hospitals.

Tanzania's PHC review of 1984 (Ministry of Health) assessed the availability and accessibility of health services coverage as follows:

*73% population within 2 hours travelling distance to a health facility; 93% within 10 km distance from a health facility. The efficiency and effectiveness of health services, though not evaluated in the formal sense, has been observed to have slackened to some degree. Sound management has been erratic due to financial constraints and*

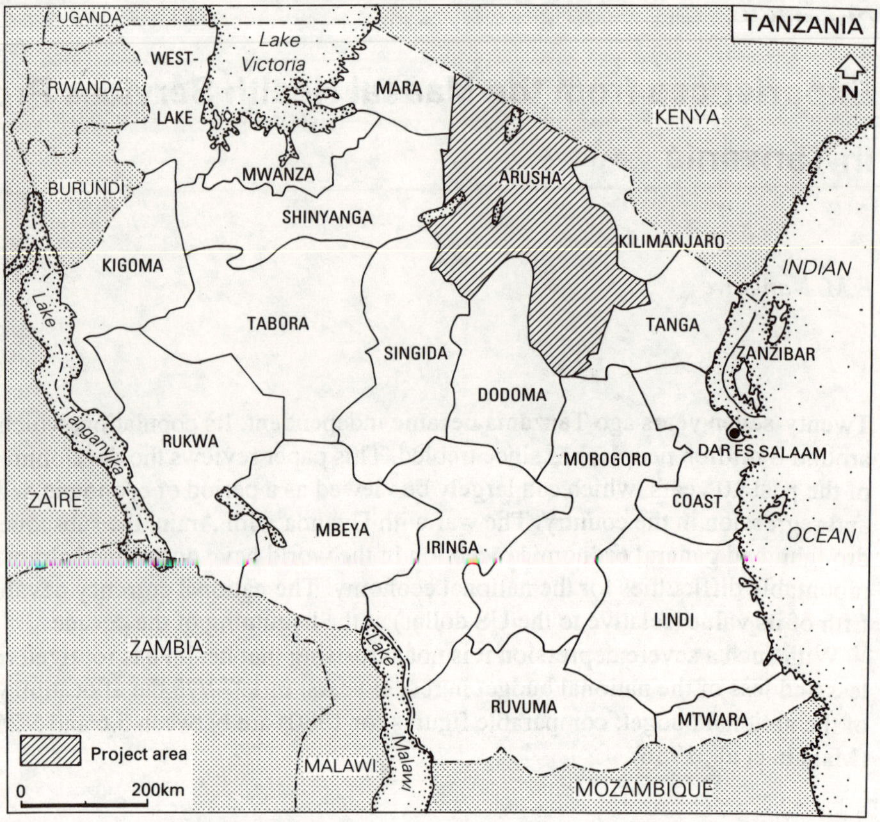


*weakened supportive and supervisory mechanisms. Broken down systems and equipment have found no ready remedy; a maintenance programme is not in place to cope with the breakdowns or the results of wear and tear.*

All government clinic services are supposedly given essentially free of charge, while private voluntary organisation clinics use a fee-for-service system. The Ministry of Health controls registration of all private clinics and regulates operation of public clinics. The Ministry also provides financial and staff support to designated private voluntary organisations to help them reduce fees charged to beneficiaries. The policy of free health services is intended to provide equal access opportunities even to the poor and disabled.

The Ministry of Health has identified women and children under the age of five years as especially vulnerable groups for priority attention. Women and children under five constitute about 40% of the population. An extensive maternal and child health network has therefore been organised since 1975. Thus operationalisation of the maternal and child health system can be said to have started near the beginning of the decade under review.

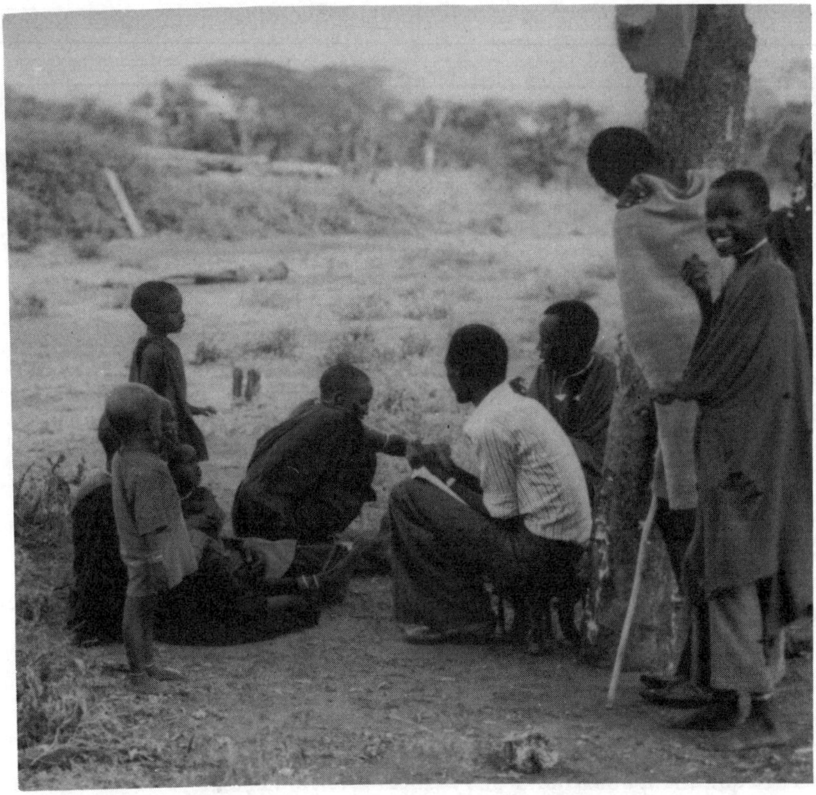

*Working on a community diagnosis of the health situation*

## The Maasai Health Services Project

The Maasai Health Services Project (MHSP) provides health services to a limited number of rural Maasai communities through a network of dispensaries. Wider coverage of services and enhancement of preventive medicine have been attempted over the past six years. The MHSP approach and structure is essentially similar to that of the Ministry of Health, despite differences in matters of detail, number of VHWs and TBAs trained per village, and processes of community involvement followed. Of late MHSP has emphasised enhancement of dialogue, promotion of critical awareness among the people, and use of adult learning principles in facilitating communities.

The Maasai Health Services Project operates within Arusha Region in Northern Tanzania. The Maasai are a pastoralist semi-nomadic people whose population in Tanzania is about 260,000. The project also serves an ethnically related tribe, the Waarusha, who share borders with Maasai districts and number about 200,000. As seen from their very high infant mortality rate (154 per 1,000), very low literacy rate among females (17%) (rates derived from project baseline surveys), general reluctance to enroll children in schools, poor communications, scanty and polluted water supplies, virtual absence of sanitation and very poor hygiene, plus a precarious ecological balance directly visible in overgrazed drought-ridden landscapes, the Maasai can be categorised as a vulnerable group of people in relation to other ethnic groups in Tanzania.

The pattern of diseases endemic in the area closely matches the poor local environmental conditions. Gastroenteritis constitutes the most prevalent complaint of outpatients and contributes significantly to mortality. Malaria and pneumonias rank second in importance with respect to morbidity and mortality. Dysenteries and helminths are very commonly seen, but are sometimes almost completely ignored, because they do not precipitate life threatening situations.

Of the childhood immunisable diseases, measles commonly claims many lives; tuberculosis transmission continues rather silently; whooping cough continues to be seen sporadically; but tetanus remains endemic. Nutritional disorders are a common underlying factor in many diseases, contributing to fatalities.

Sexually transmitted diseases (especially gonorrhoea) are the presumed cause of the infertility encountered fairly frequently amongst Maasai women. AIDS is a recognised entity in some communities. A major cause of blindness is trachoma; transmission of infection amongst children in the homesteads approaches 100%. Bacterial conjunctivitis is widespread. Anthropozoönoses such as anthrax are also fairly common.

The distribution of health facilities in the project area is largely scanty. Arumeru district, where the Waarusha live, has one hospital/health centre bed per 1,800 people and one health facility per 9,100 population. The health facility to population ratio in the pastoralist area is 1 health facility: 4,100 people.

District hospitals constitute the referral points for peripheral health centres and dispensaries, but the system faces inadequacies of transportation, poor road conditions and insufficiencies of equipment and vital drugs to meet referral needs.

The sections of the population most afflicted by high morbidity and mortality are children under five and women (together, about 40% of the total population). Their well-being and survival greatly depend on well-functioning health services and referral facilities. The preventable nature of most problems that affect these sections of the population, and the role of women in child rearing in these communities, caused the MHSP to give priority to women beneficiaries as a focus for project activities. The emphasis in all project sites is on enlisting women for training and learning, using women's study groups, traditional birth attendants and/or other social groups that bring women together.

As a result of this emphasis women, a traditionally degraded, oppressed and overworked people amongst the Maasai, have been able to take on new roles. They now participate actively in health dialogue, health promotion, and teaching other women hygiene, child care and disease prevention. Confidence, a sense of critical awareness, and a drive to redress development problems have been imparted to this demeaned gender, which in the past could never even dream of sitting in the same meeting with men and debating an issue together. Women are now leading the way in most health development activities on the project sites.

It is noteworthy that neither government services nor MHSP have tried to go further in classifying and identifying other vulnerable groups for priority or special attention. The disabled, the poorest of the poor and the unemployed may receive services, but more by chance than because of a deliberately organised programme. The greatly extended service structure, however, provides a ready framework within which a programme for vulnerable groups can now be worked out.

*Goals*

The MHSP was conceived in 1978 as a community health promotion activity aimed at combatting common preventable illnesses and providing first aid care to families in remote Maasai communities. The goals and objectives defined initially were non-specific and rather ambitious. These goals were reformulated when project activities began in 1982:

- to improve the quality of health and medical care provided by diocesan (then synodical) dispensaries;
- to train up to 72 village health workers for village communities surrounding the dispensaries;
- to promote collaboration and cooperation between health staff and traditional birth attendants (TBAs);
- to train key dispensary staff as trainers and supervisors of village health workers and as coordinators of the community based health programme;
- to promote maternal and child health services at all diocesan dispensaries;
- to enhance community outreach and community participation in the health activities.

The overall goal was to establish a community based care programme at each of the then seven dispensaries of the diocese within a period of three years. This goal was later widened to cover 272 Lutheran Church congregations in Arusha beyond the initial three years.

The project began in 1988 with an operational coverage of 42 villages in 4 districts. Working within renewable 3 year funding periods, the project tries to enhance local staff and community capabilities for running community health activities on a continuing basis. The aim is to gradually phase out external funding for recurrent and routine type activities.

The project receives funds from the Lutheran World Federation, based in Geneva. The first funding period ended in 1985 but operational time lags created considerable overlap with the second, current, funding period. Through use of seconded staff, the project also receives salary subsidies from the Government of Tanzania, Ministry of Health.

*Activities*

*Village surveys.* The primary aim of this activity is to establish baseline studies on health status of communities. Information gathered is analysed and fed back to communities, in addition to being used for programme replanning.

*Community involvement.* The MHSP begins activities in any given village community by holding a number of sensitisation meetings. Discussions are started by posing a given existing problem to the community. The object is to get the villagers to analyse and find a way of solving existing problems.

Participatory communication is used to animate meetings, ensuring contributions from the majority of villagers in attendance. Numerous examples of community participation have been recorded by the project. A few examples:

• villager contributions of food to support VHWs during training;
• villager contributions of kerosene to run refrigerators for vaccines;
• village selection of VHWs for training and some provision of supportive remuneration to VHWs;
• increased collaboration with TBAs in promotion of safe deliveries;
• villager participation in outreach maternal and child health services, leading to increased coverage of these services;
• community organisation and capital funding of income generating projects to support VHWs;
• community collaboration with dispensary staff to train additional VHWs.

*Preparation of training materials.* A training manual for VHWs was prepared, detailing tasks and essential ideas for home visiting, maternal and child health, environmental health, first aid treatment and prevention of common communicable illnesses, child spacing, and community development. The manual has been refined now and then according to experience gained from use in the field. Notes have been compiled to guide TBA training, and have proved useful in forums with the TBAs. Trainers emphasise the use of participatory teaching methods in favour of didactic techniques. Hence dramas, songs, stories, pictures or objects are often used to introduce themes or put messages across.

*Training of village health workers.* Training follows a decentralised mode, alternating theoretical classes with practicals. The total duration of training was about 9 months in the early years of the project; this has now decreased to about 2 months. Of the 107 VWHs thus far trained, 88 are active. Dropouts from training are less significant than dropouts after training. This activity has received the largest investment in time and money, as if it were the sole and crucial means of rendering communities healthy!

Training is currently being implemented at 14 sites (total VHWs trained plus those currently in training number 294).

*Training of traditional birth attendants.* This is also a decentralised activity, involving an exchange of experiences between project staff and TBAs. So far 109 TBAs have received such training, at 6 sites.

*Training of trainers.* MHSP has given such training a fairly consistent treatment, with on average one to two seminars per annum. The project presently deploys 16 trained trainers in the field. The number could have been greater, but attrition has always played its limiting role.

Skills imparted consisted initially of teaching and training methods, team building, development of training materials and lesson planning. This was followed by development of appropriate learning objectives and training in workshop organisation skills.

Record keeping, documentation and logistics management are taught in 'learning by doing' situations.
In more recent years, attention has shifted to communication skills, adult learning methods and programme planning and management. Surveying and evaluation skills have been at best cursorily treated. Of late, trainers' seminars have been as participatory as possible. This has led to a great rekindling of interest and hope amongst programme staff. MHSP experience documents that local staff are best suited and more appropriate for CBHC work. Language barriers, a rush for quick results, and cultural barriers are some of the factors that need to be weighed carefully in considering expatriate personnel roles in CBHC.

*Dispensary staff refresher courses.* The MHSP has pulled together a team of trainers to implement training for community health agents in rural localities. One concern of the initiators was long term project sustainability. In a bid to set up a system which will eventually ensure that the project can be weaned away from dependence on external funding, the idea of new training for dispensary staff emerged. Dispensaries constitute a permanent, locally funded resource within immediate reach of communities.

Staff have been trained to enhance clinical skills in treating common local diseases, strengthen knowledge of preventive medicine, establish rational prescribing, and provide orientation to management and supervision of community health.

Curative health services continue to be favoured over preventive health services, even though great efforts have been made to sensitise staff to prevention-oriented activities.

*Supervision and support.* Regular visits are made to supervise and support the trained agents with requisite inputs. The content of this supervision is gradually improving; logistic constraints have however made the implementation of good quality supervision a formidable task. All project sites currently receive supervision every two months on average.

The geographical distribution of project sites presents a special challenge for supervision and support from headquarters. In fact it suggests the whole effort has been too ambitious. Since the inception of the project, staff have received supervisory visits positively. The effects of supervision on community members, community leaders' performance, and staff performance have not been studied, but generally a certain atmosphere has been created.

*Monitoring and evaluation.* The main methods used for monitoring and evaluation are project reporting forms, plus verbal reporting and review at weekly or monthly action planning forums.

Project reporting forms include a village health worker biographical form, family visiting form, family census record, maternal and child health records, community health worker supervisory record and programme site supervisory record. Dispensaries submit monthly reports on diseases and patient statistics, maternal and child health and immunisation statistics, drug stock and order returns, financial accounts and a report on progress and problems of the community health programme.

Feedback on issues arising from these reports is given either upon submission or later, during supervisory visits.
A formal evaluation has not yet been conducted. Programme staff can be said to be doing evaluations during their frequent reviews of performance and at the forum instituted at the end of all seminars for training of trainers, to allow the exchange of experiences. Further, the project receives numerous visitors, some of whom give formal or informal feedback of their observations and suggestions for improvement. At the beginning and end of all training sessions, formal evaluation of trainees takes place. Baseline surveys conducted in communities when activities commence have provided information that has been used to indicate change at the end of training and during the operational phase.

The project is steadily picking up age and momentum; it has now been in operation for six years, with the achievements outlined in Table 1.

Table 1. Programme achievements

| | |
|---|---|
| Operational villages | 42 |
| Population in operational area | 85,000 |
| Trainers trained | 16 |
| Village health workers trained or in training | 294 |
| Traditional birth attendants trained | 109 |
| Health committees trained | 6 |

*Project management*
In the initiation phase MHSP used a participatory team approach to planning, implementation and baseline study. Emphasis was on learning by doing and flexibility to change, based on lessons learned from fieldwork. Recent changes in top leadership have not brought drastic changes in these initial strategies and approaches, but the nature of participatory management being practiced appears to limit 'total' participation: this of course has advantages and a share of disadvantages. Advocates of a 'totally participatory' approach prefer programme leaders to face participants with a blank agenda, and to develop the agenda together. The result is a high degree of commitment and motivation to action due to participants' ownership of the agenda; the risk however is a chaotic meeting, if the leader is not sensitive enough to help the forum formulate issues logically and in sequence, offering support, exercising a degree of supervision and encouraging participation in project activities (such as contributing kerosene for storing vaccines). In the MHSP, communities also participated in problem listing, but were not part of setting objectives or goals. This explains why project staff and communities have different perceptions, visions, and goals regarding the project despite many meetings conducted to enlist community involvement and participation.

*Staff.* One missionary public health doctor, the only expatriate, currently holds a leadership role on a trial basis. The central core team includes five trained trainers - two male and three female. One of the trainers performs the function of project coordination; office management and documentation is addressed by a sixth staff member, who is male; he is assisted by a female office typist. In all, the project has four female and four male staff, including the expatriate.

The public health doctor provides project leadership in terms of planning and management. The coordinator addresses activity time schedules and synchronises operational plans, in addition to participating in training activities. Trainers provide training to CHWs and traditional birth attendants. They also prepare key dispensary staff to become trainers and supervisors of the CHWs and TBAs. Trainers split up into two teams that are assigned different sites for training and supervision. On supervisory visits they help dispensary staff with programme management, training and supervision.

*Training and supervision.* As listed above, MHSP training activities comprise training of trainers, village health workers and traditional birth attendants. Training of village health committees has just begun. The need to involve 'all for health' has opened up yet another dimension that is wanting in training: training leaders on various levels. Cooperation and active support from leaders have often been scanty, presumably because they have mostly been given cursory attention rather than intensive orientation cum training. As a result, depth of programme appreciation, motivation and commitment have often not been achieved among leaders. However, thus far training has been the strongest component of MHSP. Training activities in the initial phase have been elaborated in a project paper published in 1985 (Nangawe et al.).

The logistics of the project are very difficult, with some training and supervision sites being a six hour drive away, or further. Access roads are seasonal bush tracks. These difficulties compromise the quantity and quality of supervision. The supervision offered is non-discriminatory: community health workers are often supervised using group methods at meetings, rather than individually. This has led to inability to pay attention to all individual needs, but has nurtured a sense of teamwork and community amongst health agents.

*Relations to government health care system.* Both formal and informal relations exist between MHSP and the government health system. Community health workers refer difficult cases to dispensaries. Most dispensaries engaged in project activities refer cases to district hospitals or the regional hospital, according to convenience and circumstances. A lot of mutual assistance has been realised, with government health services giving the project adequate and sound ground for future sustenance, independent of external donor inputs. Dispensaries are regularly supplied with drugs from the Essential Drugs Programme. Visits from district and regional government officials do facilitate close interaction and guidance.

## Issues

### *Women and health*

In Maasailand women are highly oppressed, and have no right to self expression where men are present. In a nutshell, the Maasai society is patriarchal; men, however, recognise the crucial role of women in caring for the family and making the Maasai life style possible. In addition to taking exclusive care of children and preparing meals for the family, they construct and repair the dwelling huts, fetch water and firewood from long distances, and milk the cow; yet they also have the reproductive burden. Training in the MHSP has given greater focus to development of maternal and child health services and women's education, in order to alleviate these burdens.

The project has emphasised the need for dialogue with both men and women from its inception, but this has often been defeated by traditional practices: decision making and meetings to discuss development issues being seen as the responsibility of men! Project emphasis on maternal and child health and women's education/awareness raising was an attempt to reverse this tradition in a manner acceptable to the Maasai. Outreach maternal and child health clinics were developed to reduce the distance walked by the women attending. Simple treatment established at CHW level with a house to house visiting mode also made it easier for women and children to care for minor ailments at home; so did the women's education package. Women are taught to manage diarrhoea (a frequent illness) at home, as well as personal hygiene and ventilation of dwellings, to reduce the highly prevalent respiratory illnesses. They are also sensitised to the dangers of multiple pregnancies and availability of contraception and child spacing methods; they are encouraged to use the methods available to them at the local dispensary.

Family planning education has been intensified in the high population density areas (amongst the settled Maasai), to reach both women and men; the acceptance rate seems to change very slowly. My subjective impression is that acceptance of family planning practice appears to be influenced not solely by the education campaign but more by economic pressures and availability of services.

In some communities where the project has been in operation for some years, women have taken up roles in the development dialogue. They have started to question and analyse why some development activities have failed and have made plans to change them.

The response of a couple of years ago that there were no women available to be trained in health care has changed. In comparison with men, women are proving to be the more active and more committed community health workers. A few examples of development efforts initiated by women can now be cited by the project; none can be cited on the men's side.

Due to improved availability and accessibility, basic health services are better equipped now than ten years ago to meet the needs of women. The services are, however, no better with regard to affordability and efficiency; here they have probably worsened. Women have no control over the domestic economy as yet. Further, considerable delays continue to be experienced at service stations. The interests of women have not been considered, more out of institutional and traditional design than by deliberate intention. Government awareness of this deficiency is increasing, and attempts are being made to rectify the situation. Within the project a recently initiated dialogue on development, which is coordinating various development projects of our church diocese, has suggested that certain facets of projects complement women's needs and can be used to redress their situation. Strategies for multiplying better milk yield cows and goats to improve family economy and nutrition will be developed; also in the pipeline is a multiplier strategy for fuel conserving and wood saving stoves.

The role of women in decision making and planning for development has been overlooked. Consequently development activities have tended to increase rather than reduce the burden on women. Also overlooked was the generally undeveloped status of women in relation to their crucial role in family and national survival. Women's education, time management, analysis of task distribution, and women's economic freedom are particular factors that needed careful consideration in planning and implementation of programme activities.

*Community participation*

Deliberately starting project activities by addressing peoples' expressed needs helped MHSP to develop as a community based health project. Asking communities to contribute ideas toward the development of their health programme was an approach that was strange to both communities and initiating health agents. People were used to being given instructions from above, and so were the agents; it was all too sudden and too new for them to believe it was not a joke!

The initiative was taken by the health department of the Evangelical Lutheran Church in Arusha Region, which asked communities to think of relevant and practical solutions to existing health problems. With inputs from health professionals, it was possible to create awareness of the need for a system of health teaching to prevent diseases and care for minor ailments at family level with the help of village health workers. The method used facilitated this conclusion: the needs and problems expressed by community members were posed for discussion, and people were asked to analyse each need and each problem critically in order to develop a broader understanding of underlying root causes.

Using this method, the initiating agent avoids providing ready answers or solutions to the problems; one provides only guiding probing questions until a consensus is developed. Community members feel they contributed the conclusive ideas. The result is the cementing of relationships with the community, using mere dialogue, rather than 'handouts'. This process had its price; a long time and several meetings were sometimes needed before the desired result was reached, e.g. a consensus on the need for training VHWs and TBAs.

It was made clear to communities that they would have to take up roles of supporting trainees during and after training, and that they would constantly be informed of developments and further programme components that would need their support. Training activities started only when communities had agreed, accepting their supportive roles.

Communities contribute food or cash to support trainees during training. Support after training varies from community to community; some give token gifts or help with domestic responsibilities, while others give a monthly token allowance, although this has often proven difficult to sustain. A few communities have helped community health workers to establish income generating retail shops; but management of such schemes has been rather problematic. Contributions of cash to purchase kerosene to maintain the cold chain for vaccines have been forthcoming from various communities. MHSP receives staffing support from the Ministry of Health and the Lutheran Church Diocese. Funds for a few salaried positions, training activities and transportation come from the Lutheran World Federation (external donation).

Working with government leaders at village level has given the project ample opportunity to appreciate the scope and limitations of the village government system from the consumer's standpoint. The project caught on very well where leaders were of good quality and capable. Attempts to enhance leaders' understanding and commitment have been made through recruitment and training of health committees. All village governments in Tanzania are supposed to have a social affairs, education and cultural committee, which is also responsible for health. The project tries to use these committees for health development wherever they are functioning well; otherwise the project develops consensus with the community as to the formation and recruitment of a health development committee. The Village Development Council, composed of democratically elected members, appoints members of different village government committees from its members. The project helps the village to elaborate the tasks of the health committee, including supportive supervision of community health workers, deliberating reports about work related to health, and advising the village leadership on health development issues.

Often health committees have functioned less than effectively because of lack of leadership training and sensitisation. A reason often advanced for inactivity is the usurping of power for decision making by the village chairman or his 'hangers on'. MHSP has started to implement a training programme for all health committees. Most committees are male dominated; women could play a very crucial role but are very poorly represented. We have, however, seen women organise into an agile force in communities where the project was on the verge of despair.

In one community women played a leading role in establishing a cattle dipping project to prevent massive death of livestock from tick-borne diseases. These women are the VHWs of their community. They have also arranged for the village to be served with an outreach maternal and child health clinic once every month. In another community, women have ensured the attendance of all maternal and child health clients, leading to an immunisation coverage of more than 80% in the village. In the same community the VHWs, who are mostly women, have started to demand rights in managing development projects such as milling and water wells; in particular they were critically concerned that projects were being mismanaged under men's leadership, and demanded to be allowed to take up management roles.

For those who had been capitalising on people's ignorance, this approach was a potential threat that had to be sabotaged. Further, agents used to instructing people rather than listening to them may continue to use the much easier way, giving clues and answers when people do not quickly give the desired replies. Indeed, when people are being empowered in a non-explicit way, no power-holder is apt to be in favour.

Tanzania's political ideology encourages self-expression, but experience has shown that poor and oppressed groups, like women, are often overtaken by clever powermongers. Petty traders and black market racketeers have recently been very active in influencing most village economic activities. Income opportunities have fed into the trend for the rich to get relatively richer and the poor relatively poorer, despite equal chances for land access. Government attempts at equitable distribution of income have been only marginally achieved. Equal opportunities in schooling and health services are vivid examples of equity oriented efforts.

As greater intersectoral integration in health is realised, one hopes that community participation will be much easier to enlist. The challenge, however, has been how to generate this integration amongst a technocracy and bureaucracy that has been nurtured over the years, beginning in school, to act sectorally. A truly bottom-up planning approach appears to offer more chance of success in creating this integration than the top-down mode. Existing traditional health systems, which have received very little consideration so far, will then have a chance for proper recognition and regulation.

*Community health workers*

Selection of trainee community health workers follows a few rather flexible criteria, which are clearly explained to community members. These include the need to be an adequately mature and established person within the community, either male or female, and willing to learn. The ability to read and write was required in the past but has now been dropped, as it limited the number of mature candidates and women.

TBAs have been generally easier to work with and better motivated to act, compared to VHWs. This could be because TBAs are not a new idea for communities. They have 'always' been around, and their remuneration mechanisms have been established by tradition. VHWs are expected to work in the spirit of voluntarism, which is probably behind the high dropout rates. The project is currently working on new strategies to assure continuity of agents in service. One option is a reduction in the time a VHW must work each month; the other is an intensification of supervision in terms of quantity and quality. Increasingly, though, we find that women are better motivated and more active than men. Perhaps this is because 'it is the wearer who knows where the shoe pinches.'

## PHC principles revisited

The principle of equity may have received some degree of attention in that attempts have been made to reach out to remote and underprivileged communities, and the poorest of the poor have been allowed free medical services. However, a mechanism for determining or discriminating between the poorest and those who can somehow manage does not exist. This makes the system quite vulnerable to abuse.

Community participation has received considerable emphasis, and is now even more greatly enhanced by increased attention to intersectoral integration.

Development and utilisation of appropriate technologies is another activity that inevitably necessitates intersectoral integration. For instance, there is a plan to coordinate with a pottery project to secure and distribute fuel saving stoves; to coordinate with forestry for reforestation, using community managed nurseries; and to collaborate with water authorities for safe drinking water. Other simple and appropriate technologies include promoting oral rehydration therapy to treat diarrhoeal dehydration, promoting immunisation, and using disease prevention programmes to contain the ever growing demand for curative services. That is, a focus on prevention is both a PHC principle and an example of appropriate technology, in comparison to the hospital.

Thus far some communities have registered reductions in number of deaths from diarrhoeal dehydration, increases in levels of immunisation coverage, reductions in measles morbidity and mortality, gradually increasing number of dwellings with ventilation, safer birth attending with increasing detection and referral of at risk cases, increases in washing habits, and earlier reporting for treatment than previously. All of these examples demonstrate the MHSP focus on prevention; and yet the results are hardly noticeable, given the immensity of the needs.

The challenge is so great and time so short. Those of us who attempted to equate PHC with CHW programmes are nowadays more appreciative of a broader vision. Structure, methods and strategies have been elaborated during the past 10 years. Advocates of selective PHC are increasingly acknowledging the inherent challenges and constraints. It appears that those favoring 'Universal Child Immunization - 90' and, more recently, child survival programmes (Nangawe et al., 1985-1986), are considering the very issues posed for discussion by proponents of comprehensive PHC (Banerji, 1986; Antwerp Institute of Tropical Medicine, 1985). The medical profession as a profession may have to be allowed to change at its own pace, while those on the PHC 'bandwagon' - including members of that profession - are supported as they accelerate towards progress. If one is hesitant it is probably better not to start, only to leave after a few years of trial and error: communities can no longer bear such exercises without suffering damage. Programme continuity is a matter of approach and interest. Among the key factors for continuity, adequate vision and process are important.

## Factors determining continuity

*Initiator's charisma.* As has been observed, many successful programmes have succeeded largely because of the efforts of a charismatic leader or initiator (Rifkin and Walt, 1986). Commitment and level of interest of the initiator are often highest amongst charismatic leaders. The only problem is that, for human and practical reasons, such individuals cannot be tied to their programmes permanently. Insight into how to maximise the utility of the charismatic character may be gained by studying the personal motivating factors or driving forces that precipitate charismatic behaviour.

*Time factors.* Many projects are either planned or funded for a relatively short period of time (generally one to three years, and only for the lucky ones five years or more). 'Learning by doing' has characterised the Alma-Ata decade; hence funding should see a project at least through its initial phase. Project plans should have built-in components that provide for transformation into established programs. Even with such provision it takes time, and hence considerable patience, to realise an established programme. The main reasons time is required are:

- 'natural' human resistance to change, or slowness in processes of adaptation;
- need to integrate new and existing systems, taking into account interest in protecting established systems;
- cooperation of multiple sectors and interaction of multiple factors are needed to realise desired goals; these cannot happen all at once.

Any person facilitates or gives way to another in an interrelated way. This may be called the 'relationship factor'. If time is not allowed for relationships to develop and mature, continuity is jeopardised.

*Community involvement.* External assistance to a programme is a time-bound, limited phenomenon in most cases. Beneficiaries therefore must be involved to answer some, if eventually not most, of the funding needs of a programme. This, however, should not be the most important reason for undertaking community involvement. The psychological, social and political effects of philanthropy often precipitate dependence and restriction of human freedom, particularly in economic terms. In such circumstances programme continuity is heavily determined by dependence perpetuating phenomena and dependence sustaining relations. While human interdependence can be healthy when positive and objective, dependence is not. Interdependence promotes programme continuity, while dependence negates it.

*From the community to the global perspective.* The MHSP has had a committed team and charismatic type leadership. Time demands on the project while facilitating communities have been onerous. The challenge that remains is how to scale down foreign dependence. Implementation currently depends partly on a core of trainers whose salaries and field support depend on externally donated funds. A major strength of the project lies in the skill investment in dispensary staff. Dispensaries, being permanent locally funded institutions in close proximity to beneficiary communities, provide a unique setting that holds better promise for programme continuity.

Even so the challenge of continuity remains unresolved, as prevailing world economic relations are maintained. The developing world continues to experience economic stagnation and/or depreciation. As a result, supportive infrastructure, including schools, road networks, medical institutes, water systems etc. deteriorates simultaneously with socioeconomic and political turmoil. Government and para-governmental systems increasingly fail to ensure meaningful remuneration of their employees and just returns to farmers and other actors in the national economy.

Such complex problems are far beyond the ability of communities and their leaders to resolve. Yet when a project meant to benefit them fails to secure continuity, we ask many questions! Consciousness raising and promotion of action for socioeconomic justice on many fronts would appear to be crucial elements that need unreserved attention.

## References

Antwerp Institute of Tropical Medicine, *Manifesto*, 1985.

Banerji, D., 'Hidden Menace in the Universal Child Immunization Programme'. *Journal of the Indian Medical Association*, vol. 84, no. 8 (1986).

Ministry of Health, Division of Preventive Medicine, *Evaluation of Maternal and Child Health Care Programme in Tanzania; preliminary report* (mimeographed), Dar-es-Salaam, MCH Nutrition Unit, 1982.

Ministry of Health/ World Health Organization, *Joint* PHC Review Tanzania (mimeographed), 1984.

Mahalu, J. et al., *The Church MCH programme in Tanzania, a study in relation to the MCH and PHC programmes of the Ministry of Health Tanzania*. Amsterdam, Royal Tropical Institute, 1986.

Nangawe E. et al., 'The training component of the Maasai Health Service Project, Tanzania'. *Journal of Applied Research and Evaluation*, vol. 6, no. 2 (1985-1986).

Rifkin, S. and G. Walt, 'Why Health Improves; Defining the issues concerning Comprehensive PHC and Selective PHC'. *Social Science and Medicine*, vol. 23, no. 6 (1986), pp. 559-566.

Walt, G. and P. Vaughan, *An Introduction to the Primary Health Care Approach in Developing Countries*, London, Ross Institute of Tropical Hygiene, 1981. Publication No. 13.

Chapter 8

# The issue of recurrent costs: implementing PHC in Zambia

*J.W. Harnmeijer*

It is the level of recurrent costs that ultimately determines the affordability and sustainability of PHC programmes. This paper attempts to analyse the theoretical recurrent costs of a PHC programme implemented in Western Province, Zambia, in order to estimate and analyse what the recurrent costs of a PHC programme implemented in this province would be at different levels of coverage. Local data and information based on personal experience and observations are used for this analysis, which touches on issues including resource distribution and the financing of PHC.

Some PHC purists would argue that the community plus the auxiliary health worker constitute the original scope of PHC, and that any discussion on cost should be limited to these entities. Without contesting the conceptual validity of this statement, operational reality has taught us that the interface with basic health services - that is, the rural health centre (RHC) and the district level - is essential in providing support services to enable the village level process to take place, at least in the situation found in Western Province, Zambia.

## Methodology

This paper presents a calculation of annual recurrent costs at community health worker (CHW), traditional birth attendant (TBA) and rural health centre (RHC) levels, which allows the calculation of unit costs per CHW, TBA and RHC, including supervision costs. All costs are in 1986 Kwacha (1 US$ = 8 Kwacha).

Based on these unit costs, Table 1 gives an indication of overall recurrent costs for rural areas in three situations: rural area coverage of 55.5%, 66.6% and 100%.

The essence of the approach is the assumption that the inputs indicated in Tables 1 and 2 would make it possible, for most activities, to reach an acceptable level of auxiliary health worker and RHC effectiveness, as outlined in the guidelines for the Zambian National PHC Programme (Ministry of Health, 1981). TBAs are assumed to perform some simple MCH tasks, for which a male CHW would not be acceptable to the community.

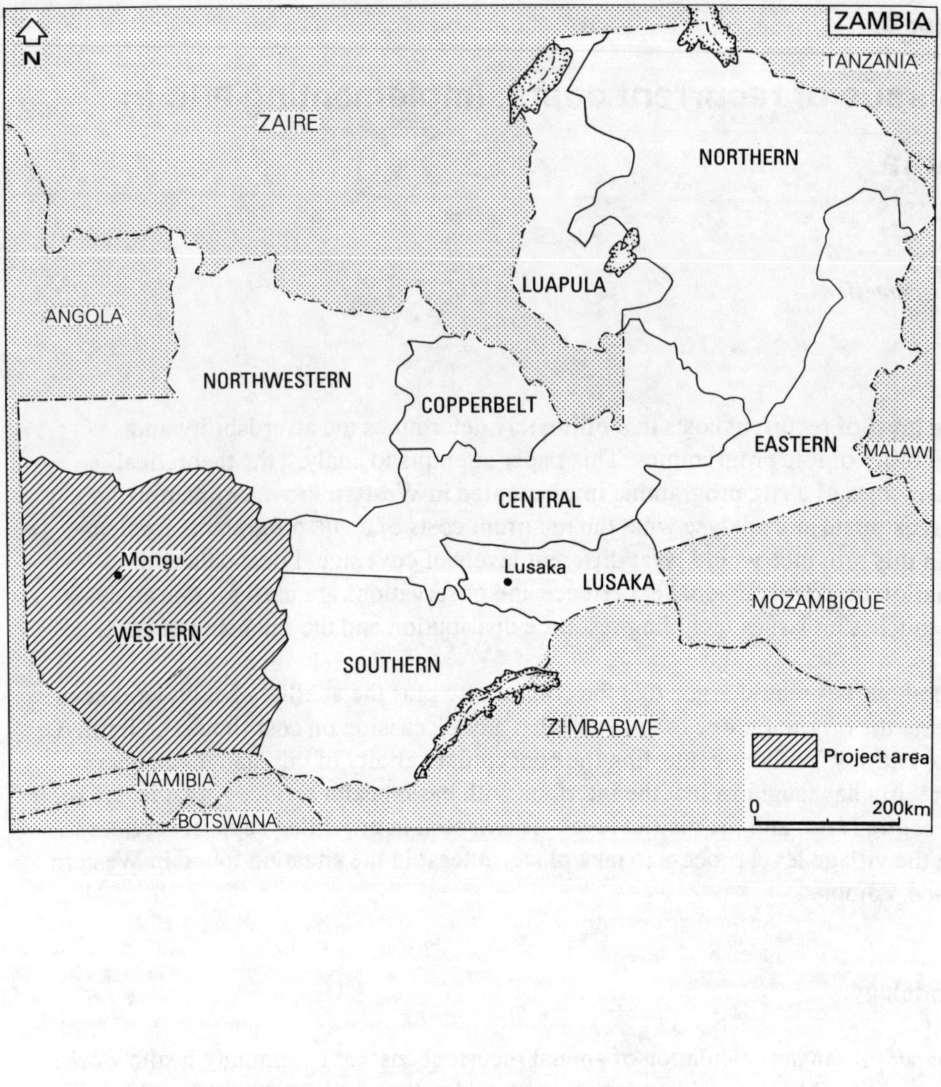
ZAMBIA
N
TANZANIA
ZAIRE
NORTHERN
LUAPULA
ANGOLA
NORTHWESTERN
COPPERBELT
EASTERN
MALAWI
CENTRAL
Mongu
Lusaka
LUSAKA
MOZAMBIQUE
WESTERN
SOUTHERN
ZIMBABWE
Project area
NAMIBIA
0
200km
BOTSWANA

Table 1. Recurrent costs, coverage, facilities: 1986 Kwacha - Population: 100,000

| Rural coverage: 55.5% | | | A | | | B | C | D |
|---|---|---|---|---|---|---|---|---|
| | No. | Cov./ unit | Cov./ Total | Rec. cost/ unit | Tot.costs | Supervision District | Days: RHC | Attrition: CHW/TBA |
| RHC | 20 | 2,500 | 50,000 | 80,297 | 1,605,940 | 120 | 0 | 0 |
| CHW | 40 | 250 | 10,000 | 4,857 | 194,280 | 40 | 480 | 2 |
| TBA (in) | 160 | 125 | | 306 | 48,960 | 80 | 480 | 8 |
| TBA (out) | 80 | 125 | | 482 | 38,560 | | 480 | 4 |
| Total rural | | | 60,000 | | 1,887,740 | 240 | 1440 | 14 |
| K/capita: | 38 | | | | | | | |
| Per RHC: | 72 | | | | | | | |
| Rural coverage 66.6% | | | A | | | B | C | D |
| RHC | 20 | 2,500 | 50,000 | 76,553 | 1,531,060 | 120 | 0 | 0 |
| CHW | 80 | 250 | 20,000 | 3,886 | 310,880 | 60 | 960 | 4 |
| TBA (in) | 160 | 125 | | 284 | 45,440 | 100 | 960 | 8 |
| TBA (out) | 160 | 125 | | 458 | 73,280 | | 960 | 8 |
| Total rural | | | 70,000 | | 1,960,660 | 280 | 2880 | 20 |
| K/capita: | 33 | | | | | | | |
| Per RHC: | 144 | | | | | | | |
| Rural coverage 100% | | | A | | | B | C | D |
| RHC | 20 | 2,500 | 50,000 | 71,633 | 1,432,660 | 120 | 0 | 0 |
| CHW | 160 | 250 | 40,000 | 3,400 | 544,000 | 100 | 1920 | 8 |
| TBA (in) | 160 | 250 | | 267 | 42,720 | 120 | 960 | 8 |
| TBA(out) | 240 | 125 | | 443 | 106,320 | | 1440 | 12 |
| Total rural | | | 90,000 | | 2,125,600 | 340 | 4320 | 28 |
| K/capita: | 24 | | | | | | | |
| Per RHC: | 216 | | | | | | | |

The simple model of a district with the characteristics shown in Figure 1 will serve as a demonstration tool in calculating the broader costs of PHC services (in fact, this model shows strong resemblance to an existing district, from which a number of the assumptions and some data have been derived).

Figure 1. District model

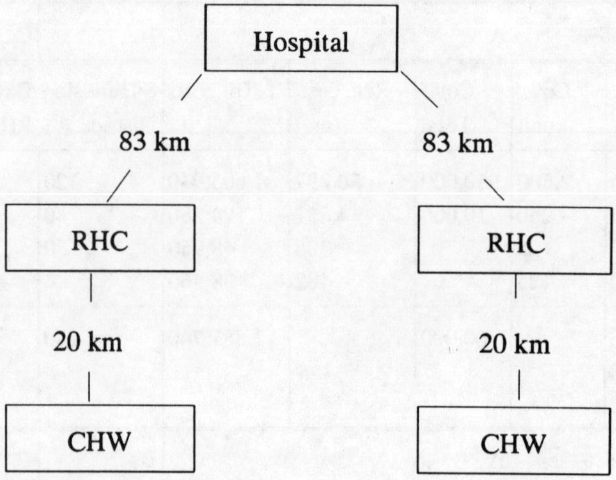


District area: 25,000 km$^2$
District population: 100,000
1 district hospital, 'urban' coverage: 10,000
20 rural health centres, official total coverage 50,000 (an average of 2,500 per centre)
Average distance District Headquarters - RHC: 83 km
Average distance RHC to CHW/TBA: 20 km.

## Calculating recurrent costs

*Community health workers*
Use of unit costs implies taking into account variable costs such as supervision and training, since these costs decrease as the number of CHWs supervised and trained increases. In Table 2 the recurrent cost per CHW is calculated for a group of four CHWs supervised by the same RHC.

*Community contribution*. In the model used, the community takes care of approximately 8% of running costs, the bulk being the 20 Kwacha (K) 'monthly allowance' for the CHW. The CHW shelter is a simple mud hut, requiring some annual re-thatching of the roof.

*Drugs*. Drugs account for 26.5% of costs. This calculation, which amounts to K 1,120, was made possible by using the cost of an imported prepacked kit of simple essential drugs made up according to available epidemiological and utilisation data. Cost of the kit includes delivery to the district: it is assumed that kits will be collected by the CHW during routine visits to RHCs.

Table 2. Annual recurrent costs per CHW, 1986 Kwacha

| | formal system | community | |
|---|---|---|---|
| Allowance | | 240 | |
| Drugs<br>Medical equipment<br>Stationary<br>Misc. equipment | 1120<br>25<br>75<br>25 | | 1 CHW kit = K 560<br>2 kits per year for 250 pop. |
| Bicycle spares/<br>depreciation | 300 | | |
| Shelter, maintenance<br>Pit latrine<br>Furniture | 0<br>0<br>0 | 15<br>5<br>0 | |
| Training,<br>refresher course<br>Food, material<br>K 15/day/cap<br><br>If 4 CHWs trained<br>2255/4 = 564/CHW | 75 | | 5 days at RHC with district facilitator<br><br>Facilitator: transport 8x180 km 1400; salary: 6x30 180; subsistence: 5x60 300<br>Driver: salary: 6x10 60; subsistence: 5x40 200<br>1 RHC staff: salary: 5x15 75<br>Total 2255 |
| Supervision by RHC<br>Salary<br>Subsistence<br>for 1 RHC staff<br>Motorcycle 12x50 kms | <br>180<br><br>0<br>960 | | K 15/day<br>12 visits/year<br><br><br>K 1.6/km, spares, fuel, maintenance deprec. |
| Supervision by District<br>Supervising group of<br>4 CHWs | 562 | | 1x/year |
| Referral | | | K 80 (oxen hired for patient transport) |
| Subtotals | 3886 | 340 | |
| Total | 4226 | | |

*Training.* In this calculation, the four CHWS receive a one week refresher course at the RHC each year, facilitated by one district staff. Total costs for facilitator, transport and driver come to K 2,255. This allows the derivation of the cost per CHW: in this case 15% of the CHW unit cost.

*Supervision.* At RHC staff level, 12 supervision days/year per CHW, each a separate trip, are assumed. Salary costs are based on 240 working days/year (including some weekend duties); for the average RHC staff member this costs K 15/day. At the district level, one annual visit by one district staff member, accompanied by driver, is assumed; the unit cost of supervision depends on the number of CHWS supervised during the tour. Here we assume that four CHWS are supervised. Total supervision costs thus come to 40% of the CHW unit cost.

### *Traditional birth attendants*

TBAS require less financing (no drugs, less equipment), but their smaller radius of activity requires that their numbers be higher, while other support and supervision costs remain quite similar.

Experience with TBA training and supervision suggests, as a crude estimate, that it is appropriate to train two TBAS per 250 population (preferably in a CHW catchment area). This allows the calculation of estimates of recurrent costs of TBAS as given in Table 1. For example, amounts of K 306 and K 482 are shown for TBAS inside ('in') and outside ('out') the catchment area, respectively. Here again, unit cost varies with the total number and location of TBAS in an RHC area, and supervised by RHC and district.

### *Rural health centre*

The same basic approach is used to calculate unit cost. In the model of the district, the number of RHCS is constant (i.e. 20); but, to prevent double counting, salary and transport items are decreased by the amount alloted to supervision and training of TBAS and CHWS. Therefore there are three different values for RHC unit costs, as indicated in Table 1. Cost of supervision by district staff is included, calculated on the basis of six tours per year, each (on average) five days long and visiting five RHCS.

### *PHC coverage and total recurrent costs*

The calculations above for cost and functional coverage (55.5%, 66.6% and 100%) of average CHWS, TBAS and RHCS in the model district are summarised in Table 1.

The amounts in this Table are costs; they do not take community contributions into account. Total costs of the units are given under A, according to their composition and coverage. For example, for 55.5% rural coverage, total recurrent costs for PHC services are K 1,887,740, with a per capita cost per beneficiary of K 38.

Columns B and C give the number of days of supervision calculated to have been provided by district and RHC staff: 240 and 1,440 respectively in the 55.5% coverage example. Of the days provided by the district, 72 days were for supervision of RHC staff.

Column D indicates the number of 'drop-outs' who could be retrained, thus incurring additional recurrent costs.

Estimates, as summarised in Table 3, are in 1986 Kwacha, and are not corrected for shadow pricing of imported components. Neither other support and activities at district level nor community contributions are included.

Table 3. Summary of rural coverage and recurrent costs.

| Rural coverage | Total recurrent | Formal health sector | Community |
|---|---|---|---|
| Coverage 55.5% | 1,908,560 (100%) | 1,887,740 (98.9%) | 20,820 (1.1%) |
| Coverage 66.6% | 2,000,980 (100%) | 1,960,660 (98%) | 40,320 (2%) |
| Coverage 100% | 2,192,100 (100%) | 2,125,700 (97%) | 66,400 (3%) |

## Discussion

*Community contribution*

The calculations in Table 3 indicate that when rural coverage is complete, we can expect a maximum of 3% of total PHC recurrent costs to be paid by community contributions.

In reality this is, as in many other PHC programmes, the most controversial and complex issue at village level. For most health workers and political and administrative officials 'participation' equals financial or 'in natura' support of the CHW. Frustration and dismay are evident when this support is not forthcoming, and lead in turn to high CHW dropout rates (now up to 50% in one District) and cynicism amongst supervisors.

Findings of a 1986 survey of 40 CHWs in the province indicated that:

- 65% of CHWs had at some stage received some amount of cash;
- 33% had received some form of support in kind;
- 25% had received both support in kind and cash;
- 25% considered the support they got 'sufficient'. All of these had a functioning VHC;
- 50% of CHWs had VHCs functioning to some degree;
- average hours of work, as agreed with VHC, were 21.5 hrs/week;
- average distance on foot to RHC was 5.4 hrs;
- average number of supervisory visits was 1.5 per year;
- shelters had been constructed by the community for all but two CHWs.

In none of the cases had regular payment ever occurred; the most regular was K 10/month for about 4 months. Incidental payments of K 40 are mentioned, while several communities had agreed in the past to contribute K 30, which never materialised. One community assisted the CHW in harvesting 8 bags of maize (equivalent value K 320) but it is not known how much accrued to the CHW.

*Ability and willingness to pay.* Reliable data on income of the rural population in Zambia and Western Province are scanty. Most sources estimate the average monthly income of the rural poor to be below K 80, and as low as K 20 for small scale farmers in some districts; K 30 is generally considered a reasonable average. This situation is compounded by the high percentage of female-headed households (36.9%) in Western

Province, which often depend on financial support from urban sources. The proportionate potential contribution of the community must be analysed in this context. If the CHW were to receive an allowance of K 240/year (K 20/month), and assuming that the 250 population within the CHW catchment area consists of 50 households, the cost per household would be:

$$\frac{240}{50} = \text{K } 4.8\text{/household/year}$$

$$= 1.3\% \text{ of household income}$$

One may conclude that this is a small amount in relative terms, but it could be prohibitive in an absolute sense in situations where basic food is often not guaranteed or available. Clothing, soap and household essentials, contributions for education and water supply, might top the list of priorities.

The argument that payments for traditional healers and the like are often in the range of K 2 to 10 or more is not valid, as these are special, ad hoc events with clear associations between cure and pay, and high acceptability. Systems where contributions were requested for each consultation have never really matured, one possible reason being that the drug supply was always insufficient or exhausted.

If a reliable drug supply could be established (again the important link with the BHS) there would still be hesitancy, as the rural population are well aware of the free services at RHCs and hospitals. This sentiment is only strengthened by the increasing burden of self-help projects (schools, housing, cattle-dips, spare parts for village hand pumps, and so on). Compounding this problem is the difficulty of managing funds at the village and RHC level.

*Alternatives.* Amidst all the 'number crunching' here, a discussion on the costs of CHWs that are met by the community may seem inappropriate. But the problem of support for the CHW is highly relevant, closely associated as it is with the effectiveness of PHC at the village level.

Of the three additional options identified by De Zoysa and Cole-King (1983) - volunteer service, community support and external support - the last is not acceptable within the PHC policy of Zambia. Genuine volunteer service seems rare in the province, but this is understandable in a marginal subsistence society where historically this concept was not in general well developed. Known exceptions were two active Party members and a retired school teacher with a pension. The problems with community support are clear in the survey results outlined above, and contributions in kind, e.g. tilling or harvesting a part of the land of the CHW, tend to be too complicated to organise collectively. Sale of drugs to generate funds was not permitted by the Ministry of Health, so this method could not be tested. Thus problems of remuneration will persist until other strategies are found. As experienced elsewhere (De Zoysa and Cole-King, 1983), one time expenditures, e.g. for building a shelter, self-help schools etc., were far easier to organise than recurrent contributions.

*Assumptions and reality*

The calculations used in the district model, with the variation in the extent of coverage, include some quantitative and qualitative assumptions and involve the application of an adapted strategy of the Zambian 'yellow book' (Ministry of Health, 1981). However, an analysis of the existing situation in Western Province does not induce optimism.

*Comparative analysis of recurrent costs.* The results of the calculations of recurrent costs using the district model are in a range similar to data from other countries and projects (Harnmeijer, 1988). But the original 1980 estimates, however crude, as set out in the Zambian 10 year national PHC programme are half the per capita recurrent costs for PHC as estimated in this paper.

When the findings regarding cost of PHC services for the model district are related to existing provincial data, the dimensions of the resource gap become visible. This is true even if we leave out PHC costs at district and provincial levels, effects of scale, and costs of water supply and sanitation: according to calculations (Harnmeijer, 1988), 100% rural coverage would require an expenditure at least five times the 1986 government contribution to the Western Province for recurrent health expenditures.

*Existing human resources and infrastructure.* In the existing situation the lack of personnel, facilities and resources, the low efficiency of the existing system, and the lack of skills to cope with the established objectives will allow only a partial implementation of the model PHC programme.

In general, lack of qualified - especially female - staff, staff transfers, ad hoc vertical programmes initiated at the central level, unexpected withdrawal of staff for other training programmes, and various forms of external interference with programme implementation are added to a generally low level of efficiency. In the province it was estimated that, taking all this in account, perhaps with substantial donor support an average of at most four RHCs could be developed per year as functional PHC units with associated CHWs and TBAs.

## Conclusion

Considering the economic crisis facing the country, one can only commend Zambia for continuing financial commitment to the health sector, unlike other developing countries in similar or less difficult situations (Harnmeijer, 1988). With the exception of 1986, health expenditures have consistently been more than 5% of total government expenditures, one of the goals of the Health for All 2000 strategy.

However, reviewing the distribution of health expenditures, one can concur that 'it is evident that in the Zambian case a mere political philosophical recognition of the need for social justice and equity in the distribution of resources has not resulted in significant change and in fact imbalances in social structure and urban/rural disparities are more pronounced now than at independence' (Cornia et al., 1987).

A realistic assessment of the political base of the Zambian situation does not suggest a substantial improvement in the future, unless a total reorientation takes place at the national policy making level, with clear and workable guidelines for planning and implementation.

Nevertheless, we can calculate the total amount that would be required for recurrent costs, if there were a more equal distribution of resources. Extrapolating from the district model data, a rough estimate of K 38 per capita in additional capital investment is required; thus somewhat more than 5% of GNP might be needed to attain Health for All 2000 (Patel, 1986).

*Financing recurrent costs*. Is there a solution to this problem? At the macroeconomic level, the only long-term solution for financing recurrent expenditures is an increase in economic growth. In the case of Zambia, with its high birth rate and bleak economic future, this is unlikely. Other possibilities have been mentioned by Heller (1979), but will probably not suffice to alleviate the recurrent cost problem in the Zambian situation.

Introduction of user charges is again under discussion in Zambia, in the form of charges to be levied in larger hospitals in urban areas. Whatever resources are generated, it remains to be seen what will trickle down to the PHC services. The same can be said of the introduction of a health insurance scheme for civil servants.

Introduction of cost recovery mechanisms and community financing at district, RHC and lower levels will have to be seen in the context of equity, ability and willingness to pay. Major constraints will be the administration and control of funds: this will also require expenditures for training, logistics and supervision.

Improving management and efficiency of existing health services, in part by continuation of the decentralisation process in the health services, is also a possibility, but requires trained provincial staff, trained district medical officers and district health staff, including accountants.

One must reckon with problems of demotivated health workers, caused by the falling standard of living and deteriorating working conditions. With the improvement of management capacity for cost-effectiveness, analysis should be developed at the district level to assure appropriate strategies.

Feedback of creative, innovative ideas to receptive policy making bodies is important: are facilities the right type for the PHC strategy? What type and mix of personnel is best? What appropriate technology can be introduced?

*The role of donors*. The direction of donor support should change; a major objective should be to build up the capacity of local personnel to implement the objectives of realistic development plans by making commitments to longer periods of assistance, including contributions toward recurrent costs.

*Health planning or planning for health?* There seems to be a common pattern in Western Province: priorities in the villages often start with water supply, followed by an increase in agricultural production (that is, food), communication (roads, public transport), better education, veterinary services, and, as fifth or sixth priority, health care, usually in the form of a clinic or drugs.

Experience thus suggests a more integrated approach to development in the province, where the role of health, the strategy of delivery of health services, and the implications of the recurrent budget for all sectors should be analysed carefully and, if necessary, shifted.

In areas with widespread poverty like Western Province, it becomes more obvious that critical levels of community organisation, infrastructure and development of various sectors are a precondition from which PHC activities can 'take off', while at the same time PHC can be an initiator and stimulating force for this development process.

As this case study makes clear, it is the extent to which recurrent expenditures can be met that in the long term determines whether a given PHC project is sustainable or not. Whether these expenditures are met is in turn determined by the ability and willingness, at all level of the society, to pay. However, that many developing countries, including Zambia, will probably not achieve Health For All by the year 2000 is less important than whether there has been a genuine effort to reach this goal.

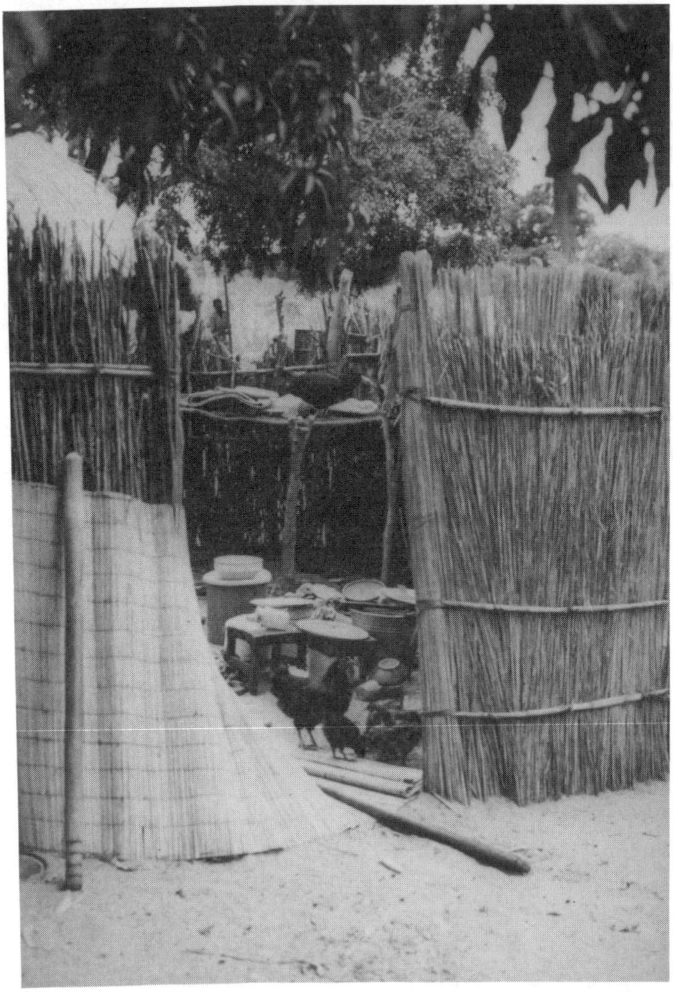

*Local dwelling, showing ease of contamination and sand infiltration*

## References


Cornia G.A. et al., *Adjustment with a human face.* A UNICEF study, Oxford University Press, 1987

Freund P., 'The politics of disappointment: the health policy-planning dialectic in Zambia' (research paper, unpublished).

Harnmeijer J.W., 'Recurrent costs in PHC'. (MSc report, London School of Hygiene and Tropical Medicine/London School of Economics, unpublished).

Heller P.S., 'The underfinancing of recurrent development costs'. *Finance and Development*, vol. 16 (1979), pp. 38-41.

Ministry of Health (MOH), Government of the Republic of Zambia, *Health by the People: Implementing* PHC in Zambia. Planning Unit, 1981.

NORAD, ZAM 007, 'Evaluation of the water supply programme in Western Province, Zambia' (draft), 1987.

Patel P., 'An economic evaluation of "Health for All"'. *Health Policy and Planning*, vol. 1, no. 1 (1986), pp. 37-47.

Zoysa, de, I. and S. Cole-King, 'Remuneration of the community health workers: what are the options?'. *World Health Forum*, vol. 4 (1983), pp. 125-130.

Chapter 9

# Empowerment through health education: the approach of an NGO in Bangladesh

*A.M.R. Chowdhury*

This paper describes a health programme in Bangladesh that is distinct in many respects. Instead of providing curative services, this programme is educational in essence. It works with the community in raising awareness, empowers people through transfer of knowledge and technology, creates demand for health care and services and activates the existing service system to cater to this increased demand.

Before describing the present programme, we will provide a quick look at the organisation that carries out this programme, and at some of the health activities undertaken in the past.

## Bangladesh Rural Advancement Committee

The Bangladesh Rural Advancement Committee, or BRAC, is a Bangladeshi non-governmental organisation. Established (in 1972) and managed by Bangladeshis, BRAC has grown into a large organisation, with 3,000 full time staff and branches in many parts of the country. It provides many development programmes in areas including education, credit and income generation, institution building, women's development, agriculture, small industry, training, and research. Health is also an important component, which accounts for about 35 percent of BRAC's US$ 8 million (1988) annual expenditure. Since 1972, BRAC's health care activities have gone through various stages, which will be briefly discussed.

### *Prior to 1980: the Sulla experience*

Health has been an important component ever since the inception of BRAC. In the first project - in the Sulla region (of the former Sylhet district), a remote area in the North-east of Bangladesh - BRAC tried out different health care methodologies, including both curative and preventive approaches. Two programmes tried out in Sulla will be briefly discussed.

In order to provide easy and affordable health care to the community, a scheme was started that allowed villagers to take part in an insurance scheme for all family members, in return for a token fee. Households paying one kilogram of pre-husked rice per person were insured for one year. This scheme was later discontinued, since

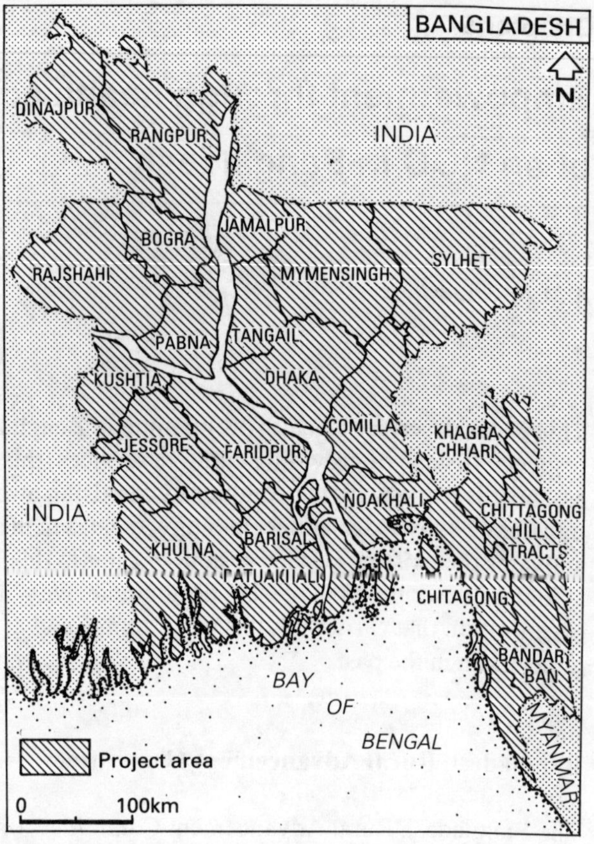


evaluation revealed that only the well-to-do villagers took advantage of the scheme. To the poorer villagers, health was not an immediate priority for investment.

Family planning was another programme established by BRAC in Sulla. Village based female family planning workers were recruited and trained to motivate and to distribute non-clinical contraceptives, particularly a pill used orally. Although the contraceptive continuation rate was quite high for any project active at that time in Bangladesh (Chowdhury and Chowdhury, 1978), the project was not able to recruit more than 20 percent of fecund couples. It was concluded that 'couples will not necessarily limit their family size unless some basic needs, such as economic, social and cultural, are met' (Chowdhury, 1978).

*1980-1986: the ORT Programme*

In 1980, BRAC undertook a programme to teach all mothers of rural Bangladesh the use of oral rehydration therapy (ORT) for diarrhoea. Research conducted by BRAC found that a 'safe and effective' oral rehydration salt (ORS) solution could be made by mothers at home with home ingredients to treat their children's diarrhoea. A pilot project in the Sulla area also found that mothers could be effectively trained by specially trained female health workers (Ellerbrock, 1981). Based on these results, a nationwide programme was launched, which was intended to cover the whole country by 1990. By

September 1986, health workers had visited and trained mothers in eight million households, more than half of all the households in Bangladesh. More details regarding this programme, including its innovativeness (such as salary incentives for its workers) are given by Abed (1983).

How successful has this programme been? In scale it is the largest ORT programme in the world. No other programme has tried to teach so many mothers individually. This is also one of the few programmes that has been extensively researched. Monitoring visits to mothers one month after teaching found a high level of retention of knowledge: 90 percent of the mothers were preparing a solution in the range considered scientifically 'safe and effective' (with a sodium concentration in the range of 30 to 99 mmol/l). What is the retention after a longer period? Later studies found similar results up to six months following teaching (Chowdhury, 1982). However, knowledge was found to drop off 12 or 24 months after teaching (Chowdhury, 1986a; Chowdhury et al., 1988). This led BRAC to review its programme. New programme elements such as media advertisements and a change in teaching methodology were introduced. Recent results show that the problem has been corrected; mothers taught 12 months previously were capable of preparing 'safe and effective' solutions.

The extent of ORT usage has also been investigated. Although the average use for all types of mild, moderate and severe diarrhoea was low, it was encouragingly high in severe cases, with up to 55% of severe diarrhoea cases using the solution (Chowdhury et al., 1988; Chowdhury et al., in press). This is more important, as ORT is more useful in rehydration, and only severe cases lead to dehydration and death.

The impact on mortality has also been investigated. This suggested a significant impact of this programme, but due to methodological limitations this finding remains inconclusive (Chowdhury, 1987).

Many other aspects of this programme have been studied, including cost, perceptions, and constraints; these are available elsewhere (Chowdhury et al., 1988; Chowdhury, 1986a; Chowdhury, 1986b).

*The present programme*

*Projects.* The ORT programme was a success in many respects. It took BRAC to the doorstep of more than half of Bangladesh's households, which provided self-confidence. Although diarrhoea is one of the major killers in childhood, there are others whose contribution to total child mortality and morbidity is no less significant, and for which proven interventions are available. These include the six diseases for which vaccines are available. Further, vitamin A deficiency is acute in rural Bangladesh (Helen Keller International, 1985). Considering this, BRAC decided to include these two interventions in its ORT programme, which resulted in renaming the project OIA (for ORT, immunisation and vitamin A). With respect to the latter two elements (immunisation and vitamin A), BRAC decided to contribute by creating awareness and demand for immunisation and vitamin A capsules and by promoting production and consumption of foods rich in vitamin A. As both immunisation services and vitamin A necessitate a continuous supply line, BRAC also decided to help the government strengthen its system, by providing training to lower and mid-level workers.

This programme started in October 1986, and will cover the last one-third of the country by 1990. Besides house-to-house teaching of the three elements, a media campaign has also been launched via radio and television, to supplement door-to-door activities.

To develop a system that will include other features of PHC, as enunciated in the Alma-Ata declaration, a primary health care programme was started in five *upazilas* (sub-districts, each with 2,000,000 population) in October 1986. In addition to ORT, immunisation and vitamin A, the project sought to cover other areas of PHC such as training traditional birth attendants, nutrition education, safe water and sanitation, family planning and basic curative care. All these elements are educational in nature and tend to raise awareness and create demand. BRAC does not provide any services on the supply side; rather it tries to work as a link between the villagers and the government system, which is available but mostly remains unused.

To ensure participation and continuity, BRAC has been trying to form village health committees and mothers' clubs. Although many of these institutions have been formed and some are working, more time will probably be required to assess their real effectiveness. The VHCs have equal male and female representation.

*Staff training*. Training for the staff is both in-service and in classrooms. Initially, at the ORT programme stage, front-line female health workers were selected from their native districts. This has been discontinued; they are now selected from all over Bangladesh. Their supervisors, who are male, are selected nationally. In the initial stage, health workers are given training, the duration of which depends on the nature of their responsibilities. Thereafter these staff are sent to the field, where they are constantly monitored and provided with feedback on their performance. Refresher training is also arranged once or twice a year. Most training is conducted at the BRAC Training and Resource Centre, in collaboration with the programme.

*Monitoring and Evaluation*. Monitoring of the programme is done by the programme staff. Each component of the programme has its own monitoring indicators. This monitoring is continuous, and is fed back for programme and staff development.

Evaluations, both formative and summative, are done by the Research and Evaluation Division, an independent unit within BRAC. Results from these evaluations are fed back to the programme. Those of wider interest are published in national and international journals. A list of health programme evaluations done in 1987 are given in Table 1.

*Funding*. Most of the funding for BRAC comes from overseas donors, including NGOs, multilateral agencies and governments. For example, the present health programme is funded by the Swedish International Development Agency (SIDA), Swiss Development Cooperation and UNICEF.

## Discussion

BRAC health programmes initially had a curative bias, which has now been reversed. This has been done for two primary reasons. First, the experience that most such services do not reach those most in need - the poorer sections. Second, the realisation that such curative services need a constant supply line, which an NGO like BRAC cannot ensure in the long run. The BRAC programme has thus evolved into an educational programme, which tries to empower the people to manage their own health, either by themselves or with help from the government. To ensure continued government services, the people will need community institutions such as village health committees, which can demand these services if they are not forthcoming. This empowerment approach is being implemented by using three types of resources, as seen in Table 2.

Most of these empowerments, except ORT, have started only recently; it is probably too early to pass any judgment about their effectiveness. The outcome of the ORT programme is well documented, and the results of a survey of initial coverage of immunisation are encouraging. Detailed research is underway to monitor the effectiveness of these strategies.

Good health will follow when both the people and the government agree to and are able to perform their responsibilities. In this process, an NGO can play only the role of a catalyst. We feel that good and sustainable PHC can be implemented only by governments. However, NGOs can play a very important role in hastening the process, both through an educational programme and by helping governments to strengthen and streamline their systems. A larger and more sustainable impact can then follow.

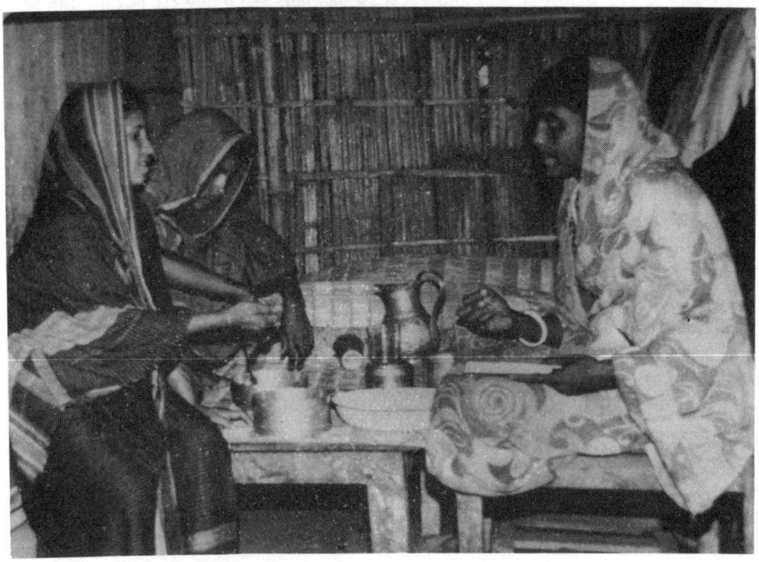

*Health worker (right) teaching mothers how to make a solution to combat diarrhoea*

Table 1. 1987 health programme evaluations carried out by BRAC Research and Evaluation Division

1. 'Indicators for Evaluating Village-level Organizations'. This methodological paper gives a checklist of indicators necessary in studying village-level organisations (28 pages).
2. 'Review of BRAC's Nutrition Centre at Betila, Manikganj'. A first review of the nutrition centre, which has been functioning for several years. It identifies the strengths and weaknesses in the planning and implementation policies and recommends future policies (69 pages).
3. 'A Manual on Cause of Death Reporting by Non-medical Interviewers' (draft). A manual intended to be used by non-medical interviewers who are currently registering vital events in different locations as part of monitoring impact of health programmes (26 pages).
4. 'The Health, Family Planning and Nutrition Programme of Manikganj Integrated Project'. Documentation of the various programmes of the Manikganj project on health, family planning and nutrition (30 pages).
5. 'The Child Survival Programme - A Report on a Pilot Experiment in Sonargaon Upazila'. Documentation of the pilot project done prior to the launching of the Child Survival Programme; reports on ORT teaching and immunisations (BCG, TT, DPT, Polio and Measles) (26 pages).
6. 'Comparative Community Study on the Safety and Acceptance of Rice-based and Gur-based ORS - Interim Report on the Implementation of Teaching Programme'. A report on experiences in teaching gur-based and rice-based ORS methods to mothers in three different areas. This deals particularly with the cost of the programme (36 pages).
7. 'Teaching ORT to Mothers - Individually or in Groups?' A research report on a study comparing the outcomes of teaching ORT by two different methods (9 pages).
8. 'A Study on Perceptions About Six EPI Diseases and Vaccination'. This report is the result of an in-depth study in 8 villages of Manikganj and Joypurhat districts, which looked at perceptions of villagers of the six EPI diseases and vaccination. The implications of such perceptions for the Expanded Programme on Immunisation (EPI) in Bangladesh are discussed (31 pages).
9. 'Mortality Effects of the BRAC ORT Programme in Rural Bangladesh: An Assessment of the First Phase Experience'. A first report on the study, initiated in 1981 to measure the impact of BRAC's ORT programme on infant and child mortality (21 pages).
10. 'An Assessment of the Tetanus Toxoid Immunization Programme in Two Villages of Manikganj Project'. This report evaluates the coverage of the programme in Manikganj prior to undertaking a broader immunisation programme against the 6 EPI diseases, and looks at reasons many women were not immunised (9 pages).
11. 'The Vitamin A Capsule Distribution Programme: A Coverage Survey in Six Rural Areas of Bangladesh'. A report on the survey done following the June-July 1987 distribution cycle of VAC in six unions of the districts of Manikganj and Joypurhat (7 pages).
12. 'The Primary Health Care Programme of BRAC: Some observations from a trip to Santhia Upazila'. A spot observation report discussing the problems of the PHC programme and particularly focusing on the village health committee, the Shastha Shebika (village health worker), growth monitoring and the question of involvement of doctors in the programme (14 pages).
13. 'Incentives for Family Planning: A review of Experiences and Their Relevance for BRAC'. A background paper prepared for a workshop on 'Family Planning Incentive Schemes for BRAC'.
14. 'Provision of Old Age Security for Sterilization Acceptors: Draft Proposal for a Pilot Project' (14 pages).
15. 'The ORT Programme in Bangladesh: Description, Evaluation Methods and Results'. A paper prepared for the First Meeting of the Community Epidemiology/Health Management Network (30 pages).
16. 'An Evaluation of Two Rehabilitation Projects of Assistance for Blind Children (ABC)'. An evaluation, done at the request of ABC, of two of their projects for blind children (50 pages).
17. 'Use of colostrum in Rural Bangladesh'. The importance of colostrum is well established in medical science. However, very little research has been done on colostrum in Bangladesh. Covers e.g. how Bangladeshi rural mothers think about colostrum and whether it is used to feed babies (11 pages).

Table 2. Implementation of health empowerment approach

| Type of resources used | Type of empowerment |
|---|---|
| A. Local | 1. ORT knowledge<br>2. Personal hygiene knowledge<br>3. Nutrition knowledge (identification and home treatment of malnourishment; home gardening etc.)<br>4. TBA training<br>5. Sanitation knowledge |
| B. Government | 1. Immunisation<br>2. Vitamin A capsules<br>3. Family planning<br>4. Basic curative<br>5. Safe water |
| C. Community (village health committee) | 1. Ensure continuity of the process |

## References

Abed, F.H., 'Household teaching of ORT in rural Bangladesh'. *Assignment Children*, vol. 61-62, (1983).

Chowdhury, F.I., and A.M.R. Chowdhury, 'Use pattern of oral contraceptive in rural Bangladesh: A case study of Sulla'. *Bangladesh Development Studies*, vol. 6 (1978).

Chowdhury, A.M.R., 'Family planning in the context of integrated rural development'. Paper presented at the symposium on 'Innovative projects and rural institutions'. Dhaka, National Institute of Population Research and Training, 1978.

Chowdhury, A.M.R., 'The retention of knowledge about homemade ORT in rural Bangladesh'. *Bangladesh Paediatrics*, 1982.

Chowdhury, A.M.R., 'An evaluation of a community based ORT programme in rural Bangladesh', 1986 (a). (PhD thesis, University of London.)

Chowdhury, A.M.R., 'Evaluation community ORT programmes: indicators for use and safety'. *Health Policy and Planning*, vol. 1, 1986(b).

Chowdhury, A.M.R., 'Mortality effects of the BRAC ORT programme: an assessment of the first phase experiences'. Dhaka, BRAC, 1987 (unpublished).

Chowdhury, A.M.R., Vaughan, J.P. and F.H. Abed, 'Mothers learn how to save the lives of children'. *World Health Forum*, vol. 9, 1988.

Chowdhury, A.M.R. et al., 'Use and safety of ORT: an epidemiological evaluation from Bangladesh'. *International Journal of Epidemiology* (in press).

Chowdhury, A.M.R., Karim, F. and J. Ahmed, 'Teaching ORT to women: individually or in groups?' *Journal of Tropical Medicine and Hygiene* (in press).

Ellerbrock, T.V., 'Oral replacement therapy in rural Bangladesh with home ingredients'. *Tropical Doctor*, 1981.

Helen Keller International. *Bangladesh Nutritional Blindness Study 1982-1983*. New York: HKI and Institute of Public Health Nutrition, 1985.

Chapter 10

# Experiences with community health and village health workers in rural India

*Sr. Sara Kaithathara*

During 19 years of work in community health, my aim has been to bring health care to the rural masses. This is consistent with the objective of primary health care to achieve 'health for all'. This paper will make clear that people's participation is not only essential to this goal, but also possible .

For about eight years, I worked with a team called MOTT (mobile orientation and training team). I will briefly describe our group's methodology and strategy and the people we worked with. Ours was a team that included social scientists, an agriculturist, an anthropologist, lawyers and health care personnel. It was an experimental work, not a project in the full sense of the word.

Here I will briefly describe our group's methodology and strategy and the people we worked with. I have worked in different areas of India, but this paper will discuss our work in the north and south of the State of Orissa, in four different districts inhabited primarily by tribal people and harijans (literally 'children of God', the name Gandhi gave to the extremely disprivileged Untouchables of India).

The system we used developed gradually from our convictions regarding people's power. The following points were the basis for our methodology and strategy:

- people's participation in planning and implementation: we had faith in people's power;
- integrating health care: health cannot be seen in isolation; it must be seen in conjunction with nutrition, ecology, agro-pastoral and legal education. This is necessitated by a vision beyond health to the health related problems of the society;
- alternative method: a new perspective in health care, in which the people not only receive but also create, by a process in which people learn to discover their hidden talent and potential and become able to use them;
- social, political and anthropological study and analysis of the society: this is needed to discover the richness of the community and also to learn the root causes of the evil which makes a society 'sick', or forms an 'unhealthy society';
- attitudinal change among professionals: professionals should give dignity and respect to village health workers and consider them co-workers;
- health care should be easily accessible to all, in both cost and distance.

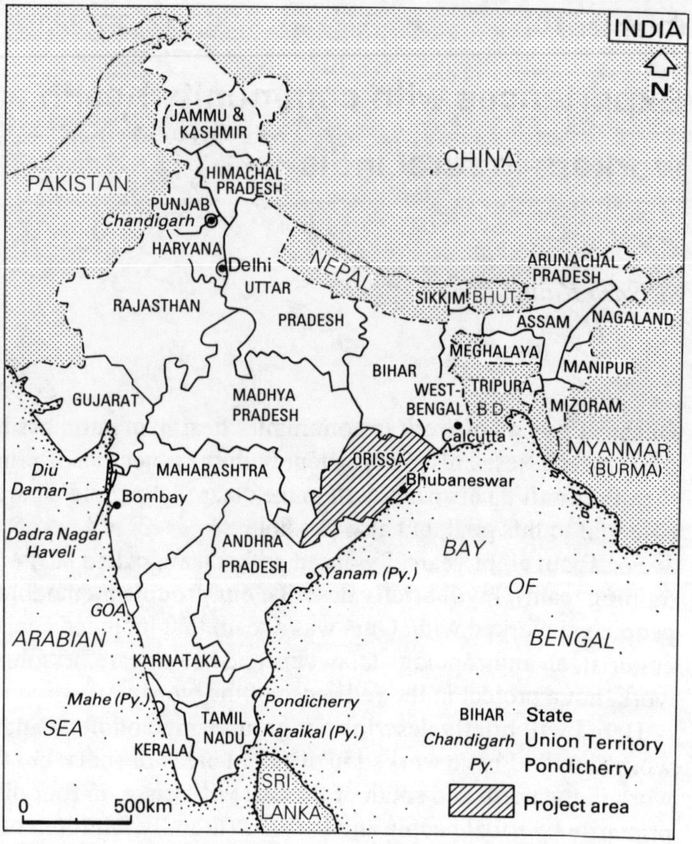


## Rationale and Method

Many years of experience working at grassroots level have convinced me that the most realistic solution to providing people-oriented health care to the vast rural area population is to train community health workers from among the people. Simple and common diseases, high infant mortality and the morbidity prevalent in rural areas can be treated and prevented by simple people, if they are given appropriate skills and training. They are capable of imparting knowledge and increasing people's consciousness not only about health and health needs, but also about the evils in the society, which are the main causes of their sickness and ill health. This approach is of course once again based on faith in the power of people who, even with little or no education, are often more capable and resourceful than we might think. Setting up such a new health care structure to give health care and people's education to the grassroots is a big challenge. Here people have a voice in all that concerns their own health. Here health care begins from the people and not from outside.

There were six in the group, and we teamed up with local staff of voluntary health centres in the area. Answers to the multiple problems of the poor are not easily available. Hence our group's first step was to enter a village and make contact with existing organisations and people. We stayed with the people as long as necessary to study their life, living conditions, social and structural set up and basic needs. We shared their joys and sorrows, and we also experienced at times what it is to be hungry. We met among ourselves, and also with the people, to help them reflect on their situation. This was a slow process of change, which took from one to three years in the different villages. We kept pace with the people. In some villages the process was fast, in others it took time.

*Training*

In health care, the most deeply felt need of the community is for medicine; it is necessary for the health worker to have the required knowledge, skill, attitudes and means to meet the needs at all times. If they have been carefully selected, adequately trained, and are given proper support, they will respond to the needs of the people and gain the confidence of the community.

We trained 25 to 30 women as health workers at a time, two from each village in the neighbourhood. While we were training one group, we were already making contact with a new group. The villages we dealt with consisted of 70 to 250 families, who were spread out in the vast forest, not nucleated.

Community participation was one of the main objectives of our programme. Communities decided and planned whether and when they wanted a health care program, and what kind: the cost, type, and location of health care centres. They chose the women who were to be trained as health care workers from among women in their community. They also formed a small committee of seven to ten people, women and men, to help the health workers in their day to day problems.

However, before community participation could take place, a long process was necessary. First came study and analysis of the society, then education, to raise the people's critical consciousness. But we were convinced of the power and talent of the people, and we believed that a small number of politically powerful members of the wider society should not, with health care professionals, take decisions for the rural masses.

We trained only women, not because we believed in women's liberation or because we were prejudiced against men, but because circumstances in India made women more suitable for the work: women are traditionally in charge of the sick in the home, and a woman can take care of another woman.

We told the people our criteria: trainees had to be between the ages of 25 and 40, acceptable to everybody in the village, willing to serve and to sacrifice their time. Literacy was an advantage, but not a requirement, as few village women were literate. During training, we helped the women to discover their hidden talents and creativity.

The process of training took about one year. There were four phases of theory and practice, after which trainees received periodic continuing education or refresher courses for three or more years, according to individual needs. Health workers received continuous support and supervision from health centre staff. The active participation of the women developed gradually throughout training. As they increasingly used their creativity, we gave them support and recognition. In the beginning it was not easy. The women were timid and frightened. They thought they were 'ignorant and had no capacity', and that health care was beyond their grasp. Through a long process we helped them discover their capacity, and encouraged them to participate. This required an attitudinal change on our part. We also discovered our own potentials and talents. I did not start out as a trainer, but I learned as time went by.

Training and supervision of village health workers was not vertical but circular, or horizontal. It was not easy, and took a long time, because the health centre staff we worked with tended to be vertically organised. However, we were able to overcome this obstacle. Thus, everyone needed a continuous training process: we, the team, the health centre staff, and the village health workers.

The greatest obstacle to the free functioning of the health workers was that professionals tended to look down on them, seeing them as menial or auxiliary staff, in spite of all our efforts to obtain a full attitudinal change. This was not hard to understand: health care service has always been seen by professionals as their right. I am not generalising; this has been our experience in the places we worked. Often professionals were not prepared to impart knowledge to a group of people who were considered 'illiterate and ignorant'. We agree there could be some form of risk involved in such a health care programme, but believe this can be avoided with proper training and follow-up.

I would like to give an example: we all know we can plant potatoes in two ways. One way is to plant them in a greenhouse with specialised techniques and supervision; the other is to plant them in an open field with sufficient preparation and supervision. The first method is scientifically good, efficient, involves no fear or risk of damage, and yields very good quality potatoes. But it is very, very expensive, and only a few people can benefit.

The second method is cheap, easily available and serves many people, but it has risks. However, these can be avoided with proper planning and supervision. A fairly large portion of medical care today still occurs in the greenhouse. It is high time for us to bring it into the open field - with sufficient preparation and supervision - so that all the people can avail themselves of it. But this requires a lot of trust and confidence in people, recognition of their creative talents and capabilities.

*Coverage and accessibility*

Primary health care aims at providing the whole population with essential health care. Population coverage is often expressed in terms of the numerical ratio of health care services provided to population - for example, number of nurses and doctors per unit of population, or number of people in the region where a health centre has been established. Such ratios are often deceptive and misleading. They express only the existence or availability of services, and in no way show the extent or manner in which these have been used. To be used, services must be accessible. Accessibility means a continuous supply of care, that is, care that is geographically, financially, and functionally within the reach of the whole community, and that is provided by methods acceptable to the community.

*Health as an entry point*

Health education and primary health care can play a vital role in increasing people's consciousness - not only about their health needs, but also about the evils in the society that are the main causes of their sickness and ill health. In training village health workers, especially in the later stages of training, we have endeavoured to awaken social consciousness and to promote the growth of a critical understanding of society. Their work in health care and health education gives them many opportunities to help people think beyond mere questions of health, and to awaken, especially among women, a new sense of social responsibility.

Such work offers an effective way to bring people together to discuss their day to day problems and take responsibility for them. The idea that most diseases can be prevented, that their children need not go blind, or even die in large numbers in early childhood, is appealing and stimulates reflection. If people take responsibility for better health, they are lead to do the same in related spheres. Many examples could be given. Here is one simple story that holds immense promise for the future:

In one interior region, every year a herd of elephants would come from nearby forests and destroy the crops in the village fields. Initially this was occasional, but then the elephants' visits became more frequent, causing much damage to crops, so that people had very little to eat. The health worker persuaded the people to have a village meeting to discuss what could be done. The villagers decided on a common strategy. Each family was to bring some firewood from the forest daily. This was to be stored until the crops were ready to harvest. When the elephants arrived, there would be plenty of firewood and leaves to light a fire every night. All able men and youth were to take turns keeping a vigil night after night. As soon as the elephants were sighted marching towards the fields, a fire would be lit. At the same time, there would be loud blowing of horns and beating of drums.

When I visited this village some months later, there was much rejoicing. The crops had been saved by timely discussions and well planned community action. Villagers had learned that there is power in unity, and they spoke of their health worker as the 'goddess' who had shown them the way. But, in addition to health workers, there must be other 'agents of change' in villages, so that a comprehensive approach can accelerate the people's awakening, enabling them, by cooperative effort, to built their own future together.

*Implementation*

In one sense, we did not work with governments. That is, we were not employed by the government; although we had government approval and moral support, we did not have financial support. We always consulted with government authorities at local level and state level, on a give and take basis, so as to avoid any duplication of efforts. We also helped them in planning health policies for the State. Government officials came to give certificates to the workers we trained. The Indian national government (Health Ministry) recognised our work in training health workers because of the national program of primary health care.

Our group did not require much financing. We travelled by bus or train, and we lodged mostly with villagers. At first, funding agencies helped us fund the expenses of training, a small stipend for village health workers and the staff of our team, and the initial outlay for medicine. Later, medicines could be replaced because the price was within local financial possibilities. We were running an inexpensive program.

We made every effort to teach appropriate technology, both in health and food production, using locally available materials; solar heating, compost pits, organic gardening, bluegreen alga to grow more food, better storage techniques, simple water filtering systems, etc. Village health committees and village animators as well as health workers were taught these techniques. Local people use simple home remedies, herbal medicines and the less sophisticated of the western drugs. Usually these are sufficient because of timely attention to the sick. The drugs used by health workers came from a central purchasing system in centrally located health centres. Once a month, village health workers went to their respective health centres for meetings, and at the same time replenished their stock of essential and inexpensive drugs.

About five percent of the sick required referrals. They went to the district hospital or private voluntary organisation hospital. These were situated very far away, and lack of communication made things more difficult. We used both facilities.

Our team was not entirely on its own. We always worked with local voluntary organisations that ran small health centres. When we left in 1985, these centres took over the entire program.

*Evaluation.* We had periodic evaluations. The objective of our evaluation was to search and reflect together with the people. This was a process of action, reflection and action. We did not evaluate to find out the extent of our achievements, but to see how much all of the people involved had grown - not only the village health workers and the people of the village, but the team as a whole.

## Conclusion

The experiences described here relate to my work with tribes and weaker sections of the Indian rural society between 1968 and 1985. In 1985 I left India for Peru; hence I cannot discuss present, past or future nationwide Indian health programs. Letters received indicate that our group's organisation has continued to function, although some changes have taken place, due to differences in individual style.

My experience with this experimental, multidisciplinary team shows that 'health for all' is a hope for the future, but it is just beginning. In spite of different conditions in different areas, I think that the basic points of methodology and strategies described in the introduction will hold for all projects in rural areas. People's power and creativity exist everywhere, and they must be allowed to grow and to take the lead.

Health workers need information and cooperation from those in other disciplines: we need to know and understand the people before we can work with and for them. A sound ecology and agro-pastoral production, as well as integrated medical care - such as herbal medicine and naturopathy - are important parts of any 'health for all' project.

## References


Moving Closer to the Rural Poor: Shared experience of the Mobile Orientation and Training Team (MOTT), New Delhi, 1979.

Volken, H., Kumar, A. and S. Kaithathara (eds.), *Learning from the Rural Poor: Shared Experiences of the Mobile Orientation and Training Team* (MOTT). New Delhi, Indian Social Institute, 1982.


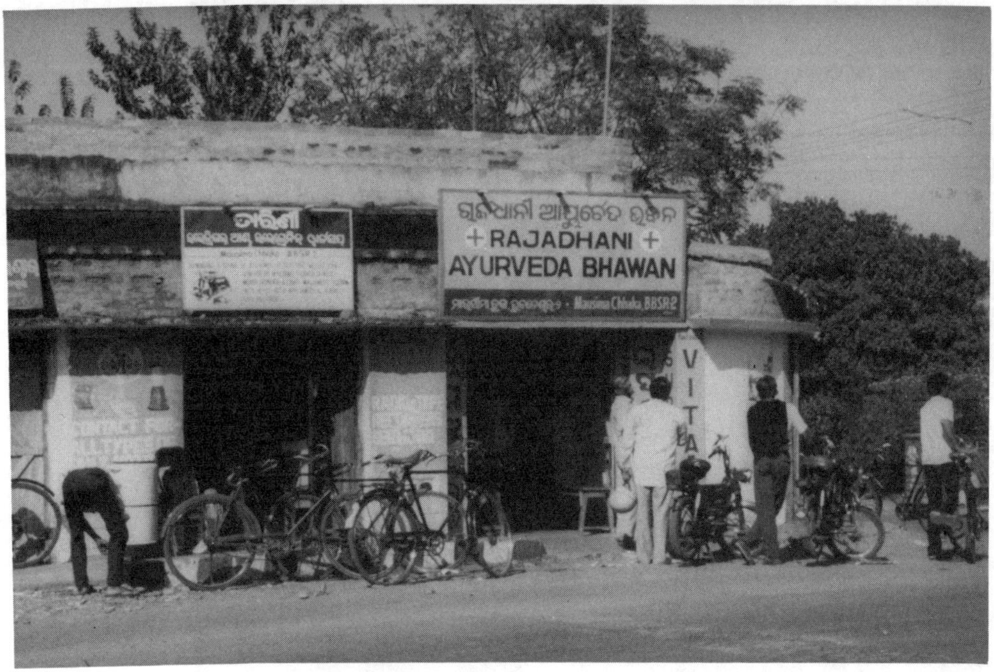


*Ayurvedic shop: traditional medicine is an important resource*

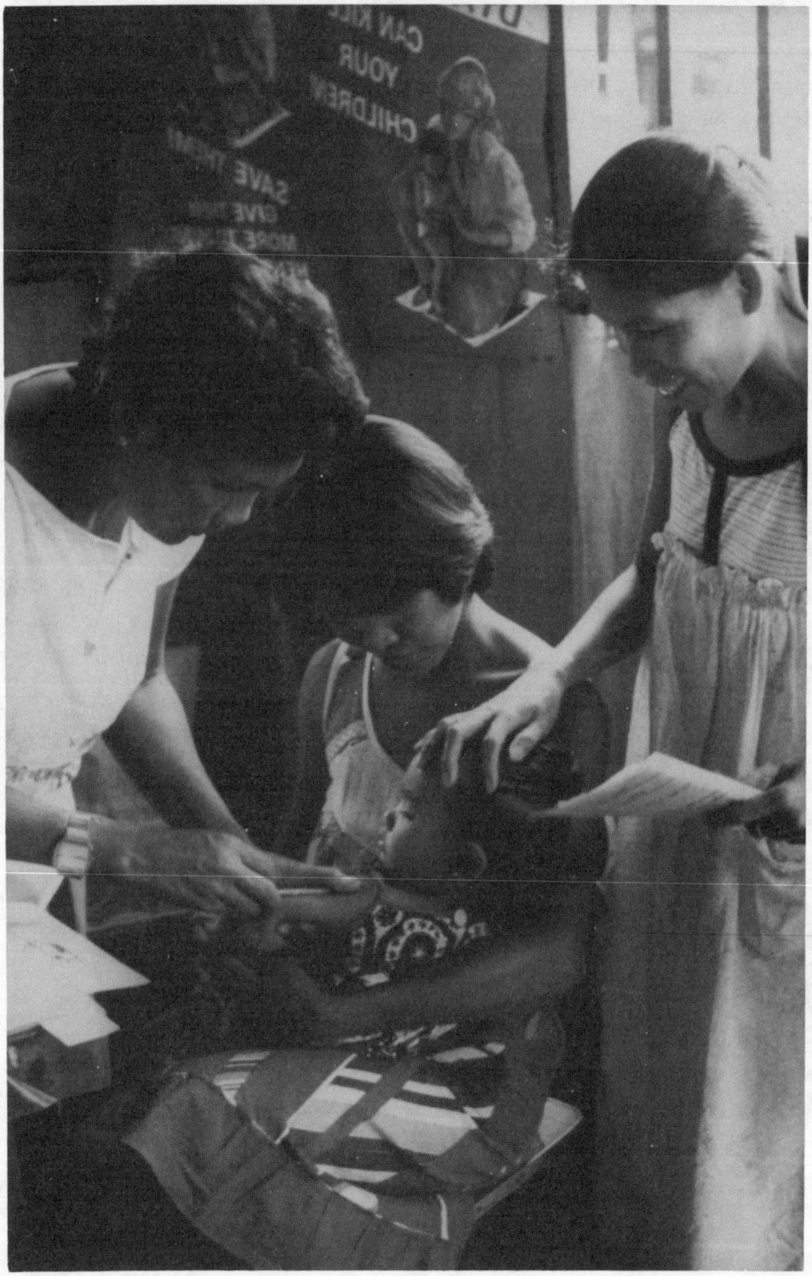


*An immunisation session in the Philippines, organised by community health workers*

Chapter 11

# The Community Based Health Care Program of the rural missionaries of the Philippines

*Magdalena A. Barcelon and Anita Hardon*

From its beginnings in 1973 as a programme of the Rural Missionaries of the Philippines, the Community Based Health Care Program (CBHP) has maintained and built on a health care approach that is holistic and people oriented. This approach responds primarily to the basic needs of the majority poor, using processes and methodologies based on the capacities and resources of the people themselves. It evolved from a process of immersion in the realities of the life situation, attitudes and values of the people, and entails active and sustained participation of the people in all stages of planning, implementation and evaluation of the programme. This instills a collective responsibility for their own health and that of the community.

As a church programme, the CBHP is seen as an expression of the healing ministry of the church, which aims to bring wholeness to life. Therefore it must at the same time seek to help people liberate themselves from self-centredness and move to other-centredness and communitarian spirit; to move from paralyzing myths and beliefs towards critical scientific thinking and integral faith and to move from oppressive structure and values to a community where basic needs are met, the popular will of the people is freely expressed, and all have equal opportunities to attain fullness of life.

To achieve this vision there is the need to develop the social awareness of the people, to build a community by organising at the grassroots level, increasing participation of the community in decision making and developing self-reliance. In this mode health care is centred on the health, well-being and future of the whole community; the community accepts responsibility for the health of all its members and taps its human and material resources to meet its own health needs. Health is thus seen as integral part of the overall development of the community.

## The programme

Using these guiding principles, the approach to the provision of health services is radically different, in communities implementing the Community Based Health Care Program, to the conventional approach, wherein health professionals provide services and the people act as recipients of care. Basic health services in communities are provided by CHWs selected by the people. Each CHW is usually responsible for 10-50 households in his/her neighborhood. They render services on a voluntary basis and are

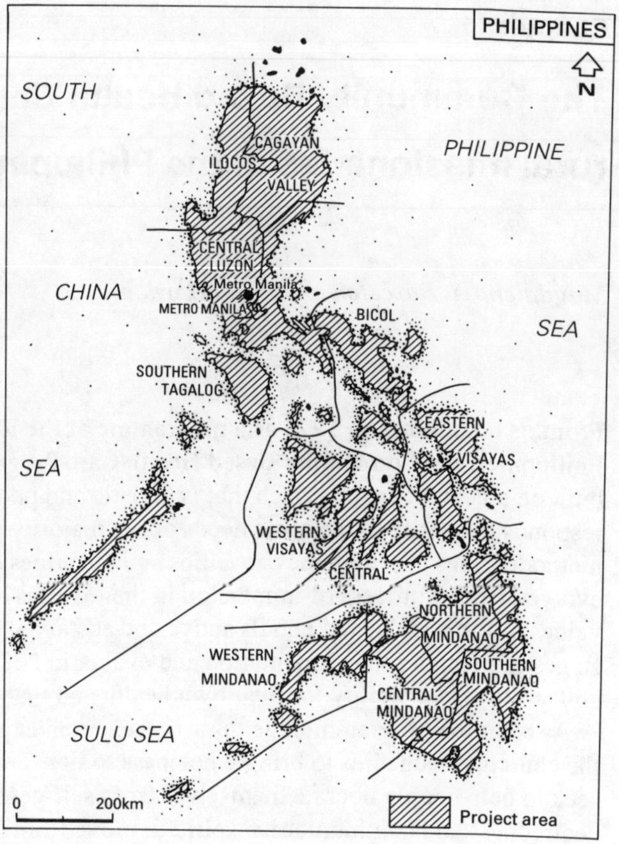


on call at practically any time, even though they are also engaged in their own livelihood efforts. Patients with diseases beyond the capacity of CHWs to diagnose and manage are referred to the health professionals among the project staff, usually a nurse or midwife.

In addition to individual day to day consultations and home visits, regular barrio (village) clinics are also held in organised communities on a weekly or monthly basis. Health professionals may or may not come, but local medical practitioners who agree with the principles, methodologies and modes of treatment of CBHPs are usually present. Experience indicates that the latter qualification is important: some medical practitioners, despite their willingness to help, have caused damage to communities and programmes when they have insisted on conventional, hospital-oriented ways, looked down on the capacity of CHWs, and refused to utilise traditional modes of treatment.

The next level of health care services are those available at the parish or town centre. Three types of arrangements have been developed by CBHPs over the years. The first type includes programmes with some access to a relatively urbanised town centre. Such programmes have organised referral networks composed of local physicians, private health care facilities and government health units. A second type provides a link with church-related health facilities such as mission clinics, parish clinics or diocesan hospitals located in the catchment areas of the programme. Formal agreements of cooperation with these institutions were worked out for referral of patients as well as the clinical practicum for advanced level CHWs and staff members. The third type was set up in programme areas with a dearth of health facilities and resources, or where coordination with local government facilities is not possible due to differences in orientation, approaches and methods. In such cases new referral centres were established on a diocesan level with facilities for clinic services and clinical training.

Referral to health care services at secondary and tertiary level is facilitated by the national office health services desk, using a network of fourteen non-governmental health agencies and facilities, as well as individual clinicians, specialists and private hospitals. The various levels are illustrated in Figure 1.

Figure 1. Project health services

| | |
|---|---|
| CHWs | provide daily consultations and home visits; organise barrio clinics |
| CBHP staff | treat cases referred by CHWs; participate in barrio clinics |
| Referral services | occur via:<br>• a network of private medical practioners;<br>• government health facilities;<br>• diocesan referral centre<br>• national CBPH office - health services desk |

## Health care services in the Philippines

The project health services structure shown in Figure 1 is a response to the prevailing health care situation in this country, which is dominated by private medical practitioners and health care facilities. According to the Philippine Hospital Association, the private sector accounts for 71% of ownership of all hospital facilities, 82% of primary care facilities, 59% of secondary and 61% of tertiary care facilities. The unequal distribution of facilities - 66% are found on Luzon island, where the national capital is located - reflects the inequity in availability of services, which are concentrated in urban centres, leaving the rural population largely unserved.

*Government health services*

The barangay (village) health stations are the basic unit of the public health care system. These number 8,784, each serving an average population of 6,489, drawn from three to five villages. Such health stations are generally staffed by a midwife and trained barangay health workers. At the next level are the rural health units, of which there are 1,991 for the whole country, each one serving an average of 28,890 people. These are staffed by a municipal health officer or physician, a nurse and a sanitarian.

At district level there is usually a general hospital covering three to five municipalities, headed by the district health officer, who also serves as director of the hospital. The secondary and tertiary care centres are at the provincial, regional and national levels. Primary health care as adopted by the Department of Health provides for the creation of primary health care committees at each level, composed of representatives from different government agencies and programmes not only in the health sector but from other sectors as well.

In practice, the effective coverage of government health services is extremely variable and uneven due to many factors. At barangay level, the orientation and training of CHWs, and therefore their capabilities for rendering services, are sadly inadequate, with rare exceptions in model pilot areas. Common weakness include a mechanical approach, in which the health worker delivers services using available means, resources and opportunities, but takes little initiative to go beyond the limitations of the existing set-up. Another common weakness is imposition of identified priority programmes of the department, with no regard for the local situation and the people's awareness and capabilities. Two evaluations of the government's PHC programme (Bautista et al., 1988; Torres, 1985) point out that this programme still follows a top-down approach. Participation in beautification campaigns and sanitation programmes is said to be strong, but barangay health workers generally do not perform effectively as health advisors.

Further, implementation of health services in many remote areas has been affected by the current civil strife. In some areas department of health support for the counter-insurgency efforts of the military (via joint civic action missions) has made the population suspicious of the motivation of government health personnel.

Thus, vulnerable segments of the population, especially the marginalised communities living in remote or peripheral areas, are hardly reached by the government services. Even in urban centres, where health facilities are concentrated, there is no guarantee of more effective reach and coverage. As the government health services have been faced with budgetary restrictions, government facilities have had to ask patients to pay for drugs and supplies, thus depriving people in the low-income category of access to basic services.

With the present government health budget pegged at 6.1 billion pesos or 3.2% of the total budget - in practical terms, 30 centavos per day for every Filipino (1 US$ = approximately 2,000 centavos) - improvement in government health services, especially at village level, seems a remote goal.

**Implementation of community based care**

In its fifteen years of existence the Community Based Health Program of the Rural Missionaries has expanded from three pilot areas in 1975 to 432 villages in 79 towns in 1988, now with up to 3,000 trained CHWs. The rapid spread of CBHPs has made it necessary to set up regional and national channels for coordination. Periodic consultations and workshops are organised.

Within the general aims of the programme to build just communities by raising people's awareness of the structures that cause ill health, and enhancing community participation, organised community action and self-reliance, the specific objectives of the CBHPS are:
• to train volunteer community health workers, elected by their own local communities;
• to build local community health organisations, which will be instrumental in identifying and helping meet basic health needs;
• to develop self-support systems for primary health care in each local community;
• to provide field experiences in community based health programmes for interested students and professionals; and
• to improve the utilisation of existing health resources (government, church and private).

A number of aspects of the programme's operations are discussed below in more detail.

*Project management*
Project management is nowadays characterised by decentralisation, with relative autonomy of local programmes from the national office. Local programmes are in close coordination or partnership with local church structures, such as the diocesan or parish service commissions. A coordinating body, composed of the national programme coordinator and local programme coordinators representing the different regional groupings of Rural Missionary programmes, meets regularly at the national level. An annual interprogramme assembly sets the priorities for each period, based on assessments of the various programmes collated at the national level. Area-specific planning and evaluation are undertaken at local programme level, with local staff from the communities participating.

With the expansion in the scope of the work of CBHPS, there has also been a shift in the role that CHWS play. Whereas in the early years the programmes could be characterised as community oriented, and later as community based - with health professionals involving themselves more and more in village life and working with CHWS as equal partners - the programmes are increasingly becoming 'community managed', with CHWS in control of their own health programmes.

To encourage this process, there is active development and formation of leaders among CHWS. Such leaders eventually become local programme staff, covering more than one village. Among the professional staff of the programme, the majority at present come from the province or region. The work of professional staff is generally concentrated at the diocesan or provincial level, and includes conducting advanced level training, supervising local staff and CHWS, monitoring parish/town level activities, and organising the referral network. Local staff are responsible for town/parish level implementation, monitoring and supervision of CHWS, and coordination with other parish programmes and structures, including the referral network.

*Community participation*

Strategies and mechanisms for effective community participation are worked out for every phase of programme development in each local area. The community based health development programme is introduced only upon request of the parish, diocese or people's organisation in the area. The area preparation phase involves generating interest, participation and support in the community, with the help of the requesting organisation. This is done via an information drive in the village and a subsequent village assembly to discuss the objectives, philosophy and methodology of the programme. At the point that a village assembly decides to adopt the programme, CHW trainees are chosen by area, with at least two representatives per area. Subsequent activities, including community diagnosis, training, health education and campaigns, and community clinics, involve the whole community through a similar process of information, education and organising efforts. Support of the community is made visible by contributions in kind plus labour inputs. Examples are contributions of food during seminars for CHW trainees or during community clinics, soil preparation and plowing for the community herbal garden, or building materials and labour for the village drugstore and clinic. However, the most significant contribution of the community is the voluntary effort of the CHWs.

Experience has made us realise that effective community participation can be sustained only through grassroots organisations, strengthened by real mobilisation and concerted community effort. These grassroots organisations or social infrastructures at the community level serve as the medium for involving the people in all aspects of decision making, programme planning, implementation and evaluation. These social infrastructures thus serve as a manifestation of the call for 'health in the hands of the people'.

In fact it has become clear that CBHPs function best in areas where people are organised in people's organisations, such as farmer's unions and women's groups. In such areas the CBHP can effectively link up with other sectoral organisations. Barrio health committees are set up to coordinate the community health programme. These committees are composed of representatives of health committees within the various organisations, selected by their own organisations. Some are CHWs themselves.

These committees plan, manage and coordinate health activities in the barrio, including barrio clinics, campaigns for immunisation, health education for rational drug use, and deworming. They discuss the approval of plans, forms of participation and roles of different organisations with their own organisations. In areas where there are no strong people's organisations, the officers of CHW organisations perform the functions of barrio health committees.

Community participation is invariably affected by local sociopolitical and economic conditions. Traditional political structures and health groups, including local government organisations, have felt threatened by the emergence of grassroots organisations. Dialogues for mutual cooperation have not always been successful. However, in many areas with strong and stable people's organisations, community participation extends to the level of effective management and control of community programmes.

In dealing with communities with some economic and social stratification, the priority target of the programme is the population sector with the lowest income, as identified through community diagnosis and initial sociocultural investigation. Community health workers are thus usually drawn from this social stratum, in the belief that they will thus be better qualified to uphold and speak for the interests of this depressed sector. Others in the village are also served by the programme, but without the usual preference for the more privileged. Thus, these other sectors also undergo a process of conscientisation and education, and generally become supportive of the programme. Conflicts are usually dealt with in a non-confrontational but principled dialogue between the parties concerned. Of course, the degree to which the programme or the people's organisations and their committees are effective in resolving such conflicts also depends heavily on the level of organisation and awareness of the whole community.

In some areas conflicts have led to a situation in which the CHWs are no longer active. This is especially so in highly militarised areas. The grassroots organisations that mobilise and raise the consciousness of people are classified as communist, and become a target for military repression. The situation worsened in 1987, when Cory Aquino endorsed community 'vigilante' groups to 'protect' communities against communism. These groups are often armed, and work closely with the army. Their activities cannot be properly controlled, and various atrocities have been reported. Between January 1987 and October 1989 four community health workers have been killed, according to the Medical Action Group, a group of concerned health workers that monitors human rights violations in the health sector. In addition, in the same period, 101 CHWs have reportedly resigned, 259 CHWs have been rendered inactive, and 366 have dropped out of training due to militarisation.

*Community health workers*

Community health workers play a vital role in the project as leaders, teachers and healers in the community. This is because they are indigenous to the community. In effect, they represent the village in the day-to-day operations of the project, and serve as the basic link with the diocesan programme and other organisations. They serve as a concrete expression of community participation and organisation, leading the villagers in health and related activities. They are also the basic elements of the alternative health infrastructure in dealing with day-to-day community health problems.

During community assemblies for CHW selection, the people sometimes add criteria based on local conditions, but generally the criteria for selection of CHWs include the following:

- permanent resident of the community;
- respected by the members of the community;
- comes from the least privileged stratum of the village;
- willing to serve and to learn;
- preferably middle aged;
- preferably holds no other official village positions or functions.

The development and formation of a CHW after the basic training course is based on the particular needs and organisational level of the community and the individual development of the CHW. CHWs with basic health skills undergo 6-12 months of practice, during which their activities are periodically evaluated. Advanced training is available for those who have manifested potential and willingness for more responsibilities and skills as health workers. Based on evaluation of aptitude, performance and inclinations, selected CHWs follow courses in training for trainers, programme management, and in special health skills such as laboratory procedures and traditional medicine. Thus, CHWs are also developed in particular fields of community health practice and for greater responsibilities as trainers, community organisers, local staff, health service providers, and health committee members.

An average of 450 new CHWs are trained yearly in the various programme areas. Of these, about 10 to 25% drop out of training. Of those who complete the basic training, about 30 to 50% become inactive. Reasons for discontinuing their CHW tasks include, among others, the heavy workload that results from combining care for their families, earning income, and community tasks, plus the repression that confronts them.

In training CHWs, the agencies involved must consider the relatively low educational level of the rural population. This problem is partly solved by using a staggered schedule of training sessions, which allows time for a practicum between sessions; and by individual supervision of newly trained CHWs by local programme staff and CHW trainers. Training methodologies using real life demonstrations, role play, and illustrated, simplified handouts in local dialects also help. Simple written information can be used as the literacy rate in the Philippines is relatively high, with 83% of the adult population able to read and write a simple message. In the rural areas this percentage is 77%.

CHWs in the project render voluntary services and receive no remuneration. Whatever consultation fees and donations are generated by their activities are pooled, to be used for purchase of supplies and medicines for the village, as well as for their transportation expenses during the discharge of their duties. Only health workers who assume the role of local staff are given allowances for transportation and food, with amounts based on local conditions.

One example of an advanced CHW is Lita B., a peasant woman who is 38 years old and married to a farmer who is also a church worker. She has three children, the eldest of whom is 13 years old and currently in secondary school; the youngest is six years old. She herself finished secondary school, and has been a community health worker since 1978. She has completed basic and advanced health skills training courses, and is now able to do microscopy, dental care, and extraction, as well as minor surgery. She acts as a trainer and local programme staff in her barrio of San Luis, on Mindanao island.

As part of her daily duties, Lita B. attends to patients who come to consult her, and goes on home visits to other patients who are too weak to walk the rough uneven trail to her house. Occasionally she accompanies patients who need medical care beyond her capabilities, to facilitate their referral to the local government centre in town or to the diocesan clinic. In addition to these typical CHW activities, she also handles training sessions for new groups of CHWs in San Luis and neighboring barrios, and supervises newly trained CHWs. In months when the incidence of illness increases - as at the onset of the rainy season, when measles and respiratory infections are prevalent - she also organises mobile barrio clinics with other CHWs. When necessary, health professionals from the programme staff, the local midwife, or the physician in the town centre may be involved.

Another example of a CHW is Agnes. She has been a CHW for two years, in an urban CBHP. She has been trained in basic skills by the staff of the CBHP, and by the advanced CHWs in her community. She has only completed elementary school. In her group 12 women were trained, of whom only four are still active. One of her daily duties is to staff the little community clinic that the CHWs have established in the community, and to visit sick people. She also tends the herb garden and helps organise the quarterly immunisation campaigns, by motivating mothers in her neighborhood to have their children vaccinated. Agnes has two small children. Her husband works in one of the nearby factories, and is often on the night shift. Agnes sometimes finds it hard to combine care for her two small children and performance of her CHW tasks.

*The role of women*

In general, the project has recognised the role of women in community based programmes, but has placed no particular emphasis on the specific concerns and issues of women. Women in the communities covered have participated in the programmes in varying degrees - as community members, CHWs, leaders, mothers, and members of barrio health committees. However, no particular attention given has been given to the role of women in general programme planning and evaluation, except with regard to programme components such as maternal and child health, nutrition, and health education.

The programme has however added a new dimension to the role of women in their families and communities, especially for those who have actively participated in the programme as CHWs or leaders. The programme has helped them realise that they can do more than just care for their home and children; they can be an asset to the community in other ways as well. Their new roles have encouraged them to participate more actively in other community activities, and to assume other roles, including decision making functions in community organisations. In some areas, the programme has facilitated the process of organising among women.

*Training and education*

The training and education component of the project is carried out at different levels: in the community, and among trainers of CHWs, advanced CHWs, local staff, diocesan staff, etc. Training courses are classified by level (basic or advanced), and content (orientation, health skills, non-health training such as leadership, and programme management). Other training activities include staff development and training of trainers.

The basic course lasts six to eight months, including 20-30 days of didactics. At present, CHWs conduct basic orientation, community health education, and mothers' classes. Advanced CHWs and trainers give basic courses on health and leadership. Diocesan programme staff offer selected topics in the advanced courses. Training personnel at the national office develop modules for new courses and are capable of conducting varied types of training.

Supervision at all levels adheres to the principles of trust in innate capacity of individuals and self-reliance. In general, the methods used include establishing students as 'apprentices' or 'understudies'. This allows more opportunities for individualised sharing of experiences and immediate feedback of difficulties, clinical case discussions and case studies.

*Monitoring and evaluation*

A need for monitoring and evaluating programme activities and effectiveness is increasingly felt. Monitoring and evaluation of health care services of the project are still being systematised, through the development of specific evaluation guides and indicators. The relatively low educational status of CHWs and their heavy workload, which results in limitations on record keeping and documentation, is a difficulty for the programme.

Health care services evaluation and monitoring is generally conducted as part of overall programme monitoring/evaluation. However, this programme has suffered from weakness in documentation and a lack of systematic baseline data that could serve as a basis for evaluating the impact of services.

In general, evaluation and monitoring at various levels involve the following activities:

- periodic evaluation and summing up;
- assessment and feedback sessions after each activity;
- regular meetings and assemblies;
- progress reports;
- programme area visits and consultations.

Participatory methods are used in all these activities, involving people in the communities either directly, through CHWs, or by working with their representatives, the health committees. Sessions usually consist of workshops and discussions among various groupings. Guidelines for evaluation vary in detail, but generally follow a framework of review of objectives, data gathering, analysis and identification of problems, strong and weak points, lessons learned and recommendations.

In the last six-year evaluation conducted by the health team with representatives from the foreign partner agency, the following trends were identified:

- the CBHP has proven its feasibility, and has contributed to improving primary health care system in the areas served, although much must still be done on the national level;
- many existing CBHP areas are still to be consolidated;
- many other areas are requesting a CBHP;
- although CBHPs have been able to mobilise medical professionals to practice in rural areas, this has not altered the great disparity in the health care delivery system or the need to orient doctors and nurses to rural areas;

• in areas where primary level health care has been established far from rural health units, the need for secondary level health care services has become pressing. CHWs cannot treat cases beyond their training, such as pneumonia, gastroenteritis, severe dehydration, or malaria;
• in these areas, the concomitant need for emergency medicine, basic medical equipment and comprehensive medical training is also being felt.

At present, the programme has undertaken a comprehensive impact evaluation, together with two other leading institutions involved in CBHPs.

*Project resources, continuity and sustainability*

It is the voluntary services of the CHWs and the support provided in kind by the people for CHWs in training, as well as contributions (in the form of fund-raising activities) for supplies, that make community based health care a reality. In some areas, families contribute membership dues to be used for medicines and supplies. Efforts of this type have been initiated either by people's organisations of farmers or fisherfolk, or by their health committees. Another form of community contribution is the collection of minimal 'consultation fees' or donations during community clinics. These are decided upon by the whole community. Income from the village herbal dispensary or regular contributions of each family to an insurance-type plan are other possible local sources of funding.

Funding assistance from the foreign partners of the project are allocated mainly for personnel, training and other operational expenses, including programme evaluation. There is no allocation for drugs or medical supplies: these are procured either through donations or from local programme income, which serve as revolving funds.

The continuity of the programme in the community depends primarily on the level of organisational stability attained. Experience has shown that where management of programmes started by the Rural Missionaries has eventually been given over to stable local people's organisations (following three to five years of implementation with staff from outside), the programmes have been sustained by the efforts of the people themselves, and especially the CHWs. Responsibility for the programme after withdrawal of external staff rests either on the CHW organisation or on the health committee set up by the people's organisations.

Two factors however adversely effect the sustainability of the programme. The first is the lack of health professionals willing to go into community practice, and, related to this, the lack of a well-functioning referral system. Referral levels are needed to establish comprehensive health care for the poor. They are also necessary to maintain trust in the programme and in the approach. People can be taught the benefits of community based care, but if the programme fails in emergencies, they are likely to remain dependent on the curative and profit-oriented private services. The other continuing problem is militarisation, which affects the work of CHWs at the community level.

## Conclusion

In terms of access to basic health care, equity has been achieved to some extent by the programme in the communities covered. The broad distribution of CHWs in these areas and the community based approach to conducting activities are key factors here. However, equitable distribution from a wider perspective - channelling available health resources and services, including the public health system, to the poor majority - is still a distant goal, the realisation of which depends on changes not only in the health system but in other social structures as well.

The intersectoral approach to health is being practiced through collaboration with agencies and programmes involved in agriculture, the environmental, education, cultural concerns, housing and womens' issues. However, linkages with these sectors is still on the level of specific short-term joint activities, rather than long-term integrated programming of concurrent activities within a community. Presently, some project staff are involved in developing an integrated area development plan for a district in collaboration with other sectors.

The development and use of appropriate technology is most visible in the incorporation of traditional medicine, especially herbal medicines, and the use of locally developed training materials among the programmes. Programme staff have also been conscious of the need for rational introduction and use of techniques, instruments and equipment in adapting useful technology to particular local conditions.

A focus on prevention has been an important characteristic of Rural Missionary programmes since the beginning of the community health practice. This has continued, with project staff constantly ensuring a balance between preventive and curative aspects of the programme components.

Finally, the fact that the principle of community participation is made concrete is considered a strength of the project. As the various local programmes assist in strengthening the capacity of community level social infrastructures, the goal of community control and management of programmes becomes increasingly attainable. Village health committees, CHW organisations and other grassroots organisations serve as concrete steps towards people's empowerment. However, the project staff realise that actualising this goal on a large scale depends on a host of other factors, involving changes in national level sociopolitical, cultural and economic structures.

Chapter 12

# Thirty years on the way to primary health worker education in Columbia

*Patricia Dueñas*

Training is a process of bringing a person to an agreed standard of proficiency by practice and instruction. Education is something more: an integral, dynamic and permanent process. Education, especially of adults, requires a two-way process, an attitude of respect, of criticism and self criticism, recognising that people, whether educated or illiterate, have their own energies, ideas, capacities to change things, technical skills, and knowledge of the world. They seek their own subsistence, have beliefs, customs, interests, organisation, and political ideas; and have opinions about what brings them advantage or harm, and about development and well being. Thus an adult in an education process contributes as much as, or more than, the teacher.

This process of adult education, involving interaction, dialogue and mutual enrichment, must necessarily mean more for the health field than teaching basic health services and analysis of health conditions, whether from a biological or environmental point of view. Education must relate to quality of life and the factors that determine this quality. This will increase the possibilities for local actions involving communities or institutions, and will motivate people to start actions aimed at improving health and life conditions.

## Colombia

Colombia is divided by three spurs of the Andes mountains, which provides great variety in altitudes and temperatures. The country's population is approximately 30,000,000, of whom 57% live in urban areas, and 38.3% are under 15 years of age. The overall infant mortality rate is 58/1000, but this varies greatly among areas. Top mortality causes for all ages are cancer, heart disease, cerebro-vascular disease and homicide; and, for children, perinatal problems, acute respiratory and intestinal disease and nutritional deficiencies.

The original Amerindian population was decimated during the Spanish conquest. They were forced to live on reserves; forced into labour for the Spanish, especially in finding gold; fought wars of resistance; and suffered high mortality rates. Negro slaves were brought in to compensate for the 'inadequacies' of the Indian labour force. At present, Indian tribes make up only about 5% of the population (10% are of negro origin, and 85% of mixed race, mainly mestizos). Indians' living conditions are usually

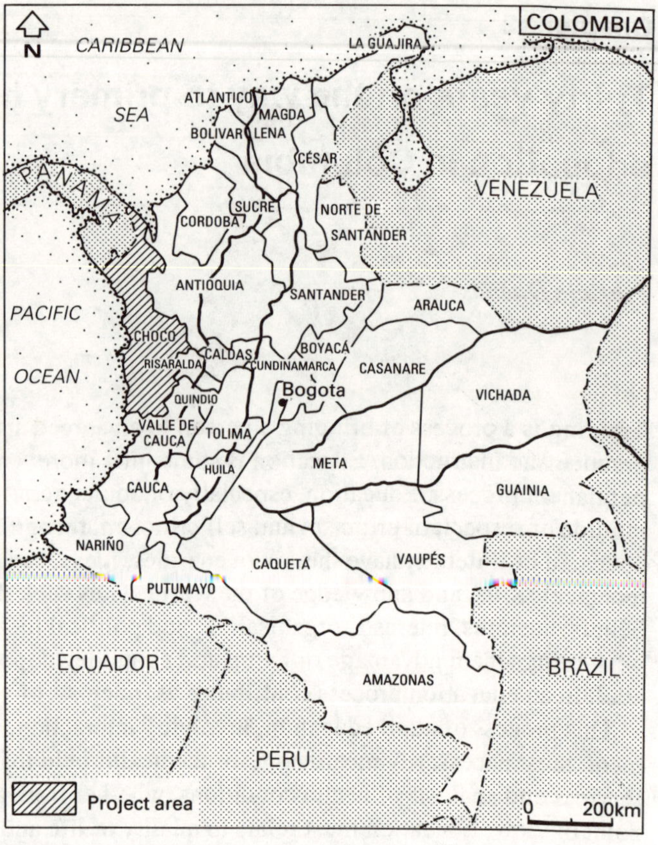


the worst. They live in the Amazon tropical forest area - in the province of Vaupès they form a majority - and in some other dispersed areas of the country. The Indians are organised into a movement to defend their rights, especially land rights. The national Indian movement has regional organisations in different parts of the country.

The Colombian health system has three branches: the official sector, the private sector and social security - the last of which is concerned with the health needs of formally employed workers. The official sector is the most important, and is headed by the Ministry of Public Health, which works together with a number of autonomous institutions in charge of, for instance, water supply, hospitals, and programmes for protection of under-fives. Lack of coordination among these institutions is a bottleneck in delivery of PHC services.

Colombian efforts in PHC started 20 years before the Alma-Ata declaration, with pilot projects in Candelaria district developed by the University of Valle. These projects included all the PHC elements accepted internationally today.

The main elements of the Colombian PHC system are: a hierarchy in levels of care; a system of referral from the bottom (community) level to the top; and delegation of functions to non-medical persons, involving delivery of health services in the villages by trained volunteers. The aim of the Colombian PHC system has been to extend coverage to all Colombians, giving priority to rural and poor urban areas, and specifically to the population under 15 years of age, and to mothers and workers.

*Training primary health care workers before Alma-Ata*

At the end of the fifties, priority in the health sector was given to expenditures on investments in human resource development (research, training, permanent education, supervision, etc.), and special emphasis was put on training adult women as volunteers in rural health care - promotoras de salud. These volunteers were concerned only with care for mothers and children. They began to operate in 1958, in a pilot project of the University of Valle, in the municipality de Candelaria. Since that time the government has developed this human resource further and further, in a national atmosphere characterised by, on the one hand, rapid industrialisation - which focuses interest on large landowners who can produce at an industrial level, and on big cities. (This has stimulated rural-urban migration, absorbed 45% of women into the labour force, and created high unemployment.) On the other hand, investment in the social sector has declined, mainly due to the higher priority given to payment of interest on the external and internal debt, and to defense (these averaged respectively 38.5% and 16.5% of national expenditures between 1976 and 1984). Such developments maintain the inequalities between provinces with greater or lesser degrees of industrialisation, between rural and urban populations, minority and majority groups, and the rich and the poor.

The health care sector has been affected since the end of the sixties by declining government investments. Greater priority has been given to recurrent expenditures (administration, equipment, infrastructure) since 1974, and scant attention has been paid to environmental sanitation.

Given this context, how have the volunteers in maternal and infant care progressed? In the seventies, the government chose maternal and infant populations and the poorest rural and urban groups as priorities. The National Health System was created, and promotoras were chosen as a human resource, intended to increase coverage of health services at local level.

The most prevalent health problems were preventable. No access to health services was available for 36% of the population, and two of every three inhabitants in rural areas lacked piped water and a sewerage system. Thus the idea emerged of assigning a wider range of tasks to the volunteer, who would receive training and a contract as an employee, paid at the minimum wage (the equivalent of US$ 100 per month at present). Once promotoras had contracts, a central authority regulated their training, and therefore published a national manual of conduct.

Prior to Alma-Ata there were already about 2,500 rural promotoras. Each one had been a candidate recommended by a community; in conformity with the regulations, each had completed at least the fifth grade of primary education, was between 18 and 40 years of age, was in good health, and had the permission of their family. They were interviewed and tested on general knowledge. Those selected to participate in the training course agreed to work in the community where they lived, once the course was finished. The course took place in one of the district headquarters and lasted three months; at the end, written exams and performance of skills were used for evaluation.

Unfortunately, this was a training process instead of an educational process. There was much emphasis on medical-technical knowledge, administrative skills and hygiene. Little time was spent on socio-educational subjects, such as didactics, production of audio-visual materials, and group dynamics. Using this schedule, with a one-sided stress on medical aspects, to train promotoras to work in the community meant that curative services were emphasised. Less attention was given to prevention and hygiene, which the promotoras needed to be able to teach.

Community health education soon became very monotonous: the promotora limited herself to repeating the messages she had learned in primary education and in her health care training. The people of the community were very reluctant to accept these messages - they had already spent half their lives without schooling, and had their own opinions about health problems.

Most health care workers did not develop an ability to relate the data they had to collect for the health information system to the situation in their community, much less to discuss it with the inhabitants, looking for alternative solutions. They considered this kind of work a waste of time and not very useful. Therefore the government statisticians and their assistants in the health care sector often could not rely on the data collected.

By the end of the seventies, 75% of promotoras had had supervision every two months, and 60% had had in-service training, in which great emphasis was put on ability to collect data. Many promotoras were rebuked for failing in this respect.

The principal contributions of the promotoras were the elaboration of a census and drawing of a map for each of their communities; rendering basic health care services, through house-to-house visits; referral of cases; beginning some promotion of basic hygiene measures (improvement of houses, control of rodents and insects); and registration of information.

Provincial Health Departments faced many difficulties: lack of candidates who met requirements, lack of classrooms, lack of personnel prepared to teach, lack of money to pay the staff for training and future contracts, opposition to the fact that promotoras would handle medicines, the low level or even absence of integration with other development sectors regarding the work of the promotoras, lack of time, lack of funds to pay auxiliary nurses who did the supervision and the continuing education. In 1979, 20% of promotoras did not have any equipment, 24% had not received the necessary supplies, 50% did not have the health care manual, and 60% had no means of transport (a mule, a bicycle, a canoe) or financing.

*Interpretation of Alma-Ata in Colombia*

With all of these on-going contributions and difficulties, Colombia signed the Alma-Ata declaration. The country had already accumulated experience in methodologies for the promotion, selection, training, contracting, supervision and continuing education of promotoras. It also had experience with the implementation of these plans and the many lessons to be learned regarding the difficulties.

Primary health care was defined for Columbia as 'The strategy which permits the spreading of health services to persons as well as to the environment by carrying out simple activities meant to satisfy the elementary needs of the community, related to health care, prevention of frequent diseases and rendering minimum services of cure and recovery'.

The main objectives of health policies in this period thus became the reduction of child and maternal mortality, of diseases caused by infection and parasites, and of inequalities in health care services for rural and urban populations; and an increase in the availability of health care services, drinking water, sewerage and vaccinations, promotion of health care education, training of auxiliary health care personal, coordination between institutions to avoid duplication, and the broad dispersal of material and human resources.

*Training promotoras after Alma-Ata.* After Alma-Ata, no important changes occurred in the process (selection, location of the course, duration and evaluation, supervision and in-service training) of training promotoras. There was a slight inclination to evaluate the process of health training as well as the results of the training itself; there was great progress in production of educational materials at central level and adaptation of these materials to local realities. There was also a bit more contact with the community during selection and supervision of promotoras, which meant that selection criteria became more flexible; this contributed to more comprehensive supervision. The daily tasks of promotoras were as before Alma-Ata: mainly curative, with high interest in data collection and low interest in the improvement of environmental and other conditions. Health education was mainly about transmission of disease.

The most important progress for Provincial Health Departments was the assignment of funds for basic training, building of classrooms, and staff training. The number of promotoras increased: between 1979 and 1984 the number nearly doubled, to 5,376. Promotoras obtained permission to handle medicines (analgesics, anti-parasitic and anti-malarial drugs, antibiotics, vitamins, and medicines for common skin diseases), there was good availability of supplies, and 75% of promotoras received supplies on time.

Some problems remained: 25% of promotoras did not receive their supplies, 60% of promotoras lacked a means of transport, funds to create more jobs for promotoras were lacking; there was a low rate of implementation of environmental sanitation services and very little integration between other development sectors and the work of the promotoras.

Other problems not only remained but grew worse, especially in the eighties: it was alarming to note that the number of promotoras supervised once in two months decreased from 75% at the end of the seventies to 60% in 1984. Others received supervision, but had to wait three months or longer. Further, the supervised workers did not receive the results of the supervision. In 1984, only 52% of the promotoras received continuing education. Moreover, the number of promotoras with complete equipment in good condition was only 19% in 1984. These problems are related to decreasing contributions of the state to the health care sector in the eighties, a preference for spending on recurrent costs instead of investments, and a low priority placed on financing for environmental sanitation.

It was only after Alma-Ata, that is to say after 20 years of experience with promotoras, that the system began to work among minority groups, including the Indian population and the marginal urban population. Many years will have to go by before the strategy for working with these specific sections of the population becomes as systematic as it is among the majority of the population.

## Education of Indian health volunteers: a case study

In Colombia, Amerindian people form an ethnic minority, with their own languages, religion, medicine and customs. They survive on a subsistence economy, and have gradually been moved from their land, going to remote parts of the country, where the land does not produce much. Here too the various development activities, including education, public services, and communication have had little influence. These peoples fall under special legislation, which permits them to have communal land and their own form of government, in which authority is exercised by a communal council (cabildo), and exempts them from taxes.

In view of these differences, the law provides them with health care services and bilingual education by Indian trainers and teachers. Training is based on results of socio-medical research, respecting values, traditions, beliefs and cultural habits and inheritance. Integration of traditional medicine and adaptation of traditional ways of community participation for use in development of official programs are included. The provincial health sectors are responsible for coordination of training, supervision and continuing education, elaboration of educational materials, intersectoral coordination, and adaptation of the hospital situation to Indian patients. Unfortunately, in reality these aspects are rarely seen.

Before Alma-Ata, no formal PHC actions were carried out among Indian populations, and economic, geographic and cultural access to medical services was poor. Black populations were better attended, but also were among the most deprived in the country.

Chocó province lies in northwest Columbia. It bounds on Panama, and has coasts on both Atlantic and Pacific Oceans. Rivers are a main means of transport. Chocó has approximately 300,000 inhabitants, 70% in rural areas. 90% are black, 8% Indians, and 2% mestizos.

Rural Chocó has a subsistence economy, based on agriculture, fishing, exploitation of forest products and gold mining, all of which are carried out with low technology. There are severe bottlenecks in marketing. Chocó is one of the poorest areas of the country, as shown by some of its indicators: general mortality in 1982: 8.5/1,000; infant mortality rate in 1984: 148/1,000; mortality rate among under-fives: 34.2/1,000. The most important illnesses in the province are malaria; complications of pregnancy, labour and the postnatal period, or abortion; genito-urinary disease; intestinal disease;

and respiratory disease. Very few people in the rural area have a proper water supply and waste disposal facilities.

The Indian population lives in the worst conditions, along the branches of the rivers. Most are isolated even from the scattered interior riverine settlements. They belong to the Embera and Waunana tribes. The Indian nationalist movement is represented by OREWA (Organización Regional Embera Waunana).

In Chocó, the provincial health sector has occasionally included a few Indians in the training course for rural promotoras; in 1984, nine Indian promotoras were given contracts. In the courses, their main problems were difficulties in communication with other participants, trainers and teachers; in adapting to the urban environment (courses took place in the provincial capital); with the learning process, because the course was designed for a different group; and with the schooling itself. What is more, the fundamental principles of traditional indigenous medicine differ greatly those of the black population, which had been used as a point of departure in designing the course for promotoras.

Because of these problems, and as a result of a national Indian Congress that took place in Chocó, OREWA proposed that the rural health care program of the Convenio Colombo Holandès (which, with Dutch support, was working to develop PHC in the province) organise a few educational courses especially for Indians, who initially would work as volunteers, but later would ask for contracts, supervision and in-service training.

In answer to this proposal, agreement was reached between the Provincial Health Sector, the Convenio's rural health care program in Chocó, and OREWA. The responsibilities of the health sector and the rural health care program were to be technical aspects, methodology, logistics and financial resources; those of OREWA, promotion, selection - with community participation - of participants, adjustment of the course to the Indian culture, and provision of supervision and further education, plus distribution of supplies.

The most important change introduced was to start from the concept of education instead of training. To achieve the goal of health education, several changes were introduced. These included the development of ethno-medical research, to identify the concepts of health and illness within the ecological, historical, social, cultural and biological vision of the Indians; and to identify the needs, knowledge and limitations of the previously trained promotoras, including their knowledge of the disease frequency in the community, their expectations towards a health volunteer, and possible forms collaboration with a volunteer might take. On the basis of the information obtained, an educational programme was created: it was later modified in accord with recommendations of OREWA, the group of adults being educated, and the community.

Participants were selected by their communities; communities were selected by OREWA on the basis of the existence of a solidly organised cabildo, which could support the future volunteer. Priority was also given to communities with a low supply of health services and access to services. The usual result was a group of 20 to 30 Indians, nearly all male, from various parts of the province, with on average educational level of third grade of primary school, 12-35 years of age, and low levels of ability in Spanish. Groups generally included one to three persons who could not read or write.

Each group stayed in an Indian community that had previously been consulted on the development of the course, and had concluded that the group of participants and trainers should be accommodated as guests, in the community house. The community also supplied them with locally produced food and the women helped with cooking. A meeting room was arranged in the communal house.

One third of meetings was dedicated to socio-educative aspects and analysis of the concepts of health and illness. A permanent team, composed of a nurse, an Indian teacher, an assistant nurse and a representative of OREWA participated in the education process. The latter three served as interpreters between educators and students. A support group, composed of a doctor, a sanitation engineer and a social worker, also participated.

During each meeting, dialogues took place on the assigned subject, always in the Indian language. Concepts and practices were explored, and comments were exchanged; conclusions were reached, doubts cleared up, and finally a summary was made. In most meetings, pictures - which had been tested previously - were used to stimulate a discussion. Development of skills was taken into account during the whole educative process.

The 21 week course was divided into three phases. For the first 12 weeks, the group met as described, within the indigenous community. Most of the discussions took place in this phase, and as much practical experience as possible was offered. Toward this aim a small primary health care post was installed in the village, so that each participant had the opportunity to offer basic health services, with assistance.

A cabildo was formed within the group to coordinate four working groups. Their tasks were to boil water, select the food to eat, obtain firewood, and clean the meeting and living rooms. Moreover, in meetings between the community, the representatives of the OREWA and the participants, problems of the community were discussed, and alternative solutions sought. As a result of these meetings and the educational process with the community, a little rainwater catchment tank was installed, latrines were constructed, wet places were drained, and under-fives were vaccinated, as were domestic animals. Also, meat for human consumption was inspected.

Evaluation of the education process took place throughout the project, in periodic meetings with participants, community leaders, the team of educators, and representatives of OREWA and of the rural health program. Opinions were expressed about the subjects of the course, and costs of the whole educational process were reviewed. Evaluation of learning was based on observation of each participant's skills and attitudes, and by testing knowledge. The community also participated, discussing these matters in the meetings. The most important criterion was the progress made by the participants by the end of the final phase.

At the end of the first phase, each participant received his equipment and returned to his community to start the second phase of education, in which each participant worked in his community according to a workplan. Within this eight week period, the supervising team paid a visit, giving assistance and further education at individual level. Also, the work of the volunteer was evaluated, with community input. Volunteers were observed to make important contributions in this phase. The most important were the provision of basic health care services, stimulation of discussions about the problems of the community, coordinated work with local authorities, and, when necessary, contact with representatives of development agencies.

In the third and last phase participants came together again, but now in the provincial capital. Here they heard the results of the supervision, analysed these results, and looked for solutions to the most common problems. They also received further education, paid a visit to institutions representing various development sectors, and evaluated the course both jointly and in meetings between each participant and the supervising team.

The educational process was supported by a manual, which served as a guide for discussion; and slides and films taken by the educators, assisted by a communications expert. Sociodrama, demonstrations with puppets, and blackboard drawings were also used.

Overall, the experience contributed a methodology and design for the education of Indian health volunteers; a health care manual suitable to their local reality; experience in collaboration with local and provincial organisations (such as departments of education, agriculture and roads); improvement of procedures for registration of health information by volunteers (data collected needed to be comprehensible to and suitable for discussion with the community); and development of criteria for evaluation of the process of learning and training, using observation and discussion.

The difficulties confronted by the Provincial Health Sector in this experience included a lack of funds to pay the costs of visits to promote the programme prior to selection of participants, and of supervisory visits for continuing education; the impossibility of giving the participants contracts after they finished the course; and the impossibility of analysing information registered by Indian volunteers about their communities. Moreover, the health sector is unable to finance continuation of these activities, which form an integral part of the PHC strategy for indigenous communities. These impediments have made it impossible to verify how conditions have changed in the communities provided with a health volunteer.

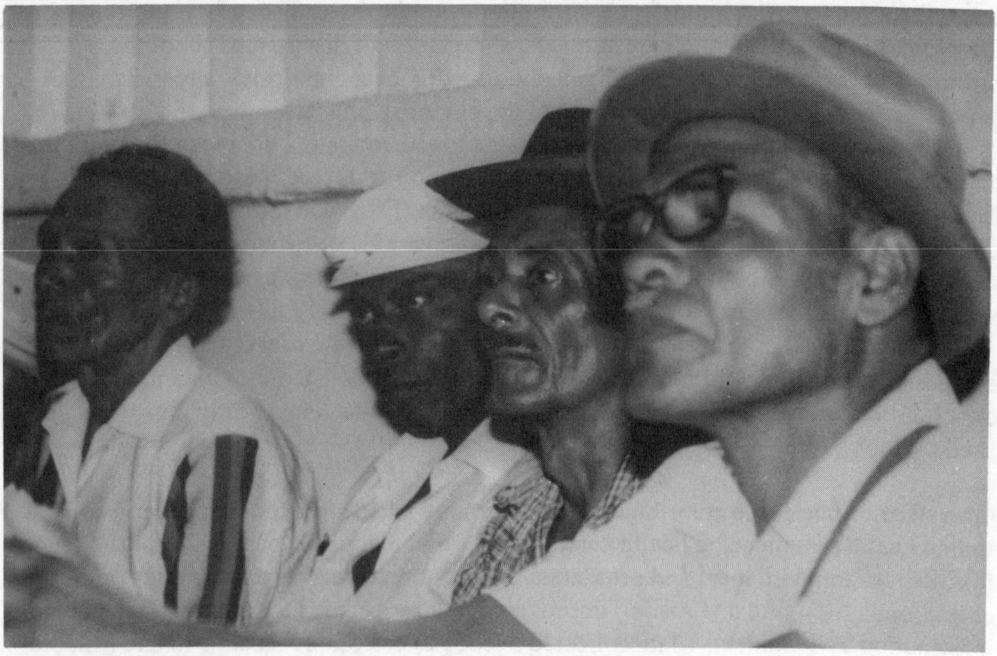

*Absorbing new knowledge requires great concentration*

## Conclusion

In the evolution of PHC in Colombia we observe that, of the PHC principles, the health sector puts the most emphasis on the principle of equity. Promotoras and volunteers clearly try to attend the population with the most needs. Nevertheless, it has not been possible to reach the target population properly, due to the persistent scarcity of financial resources - a result of the decreasing support of the government and others to the health sector, and of the low priority given to expenditures as investments.

However, even if promotoras and volunteers were to reach the target population, equity in provision of health care services would hardly bring about equal health conditions for the Colombian population, because of inequalities in living conditions. Differences in health status can only be changed if government interventions toward reduction of inequality in living conditions are integrated. In Colombia, achievement of this goal is constrained by poor coordination among sectors, and by low community participation in interventions.

Educating health workers, instead of training, would contribute to increases in community participation, at least in health interventions; and to more coordination among intersectoral activities. This would provide not only the benefits of delivery of basic health services, but also a health worker able to establish a dialogue with his community - that is, attending not only to morbidity, but also to a two-way process in which problems are discussed and solved.

To allow for this, a careful review of the Colombian interpretation of PHC is needed. PHC should not focus only on health services coverage and environmental sanitation. It should not be aimed only at prevention, cure and rehabilitation of prevalent diseases. The concept of PHC should reflect a wider concept of health, which stresses the importance of well being, and which emphasises intersectoral cooperation, community participation and appropriate technology. Further, the Ministry of Health should look for new financial resources, to make spending for investment possible.

Experiences such as the education of Indian health volunteers offer a design in which the goal is *education*. This differs from the Colombian *training* experience, because it does not restrict the practice of community health workers to disease prevention, cure and rehabilitation. It also includes great efforts to achieve well being.

There are other differences: the Chocó experience started from a profound knowledge of community characteristics. Active participation of organisations, volunteers, educators and community took place throughout the education process. This process was designed in accord with local characteristics, and involved volunteers in looking, with their communities, for solutions to their problems; and, finally, in the most important aspect of the course: the emphasis on the social context.

For the future, Colombia faces the great challenge of dealing with health problems in an integrated way, focusing on education, instead of training, in health. To take up this challenge, the country requires a national policy focusing on social well being, assigning the larger part of its resources to those most in need, and reducing inequalities in quality of life.

# Appendix

## Declaration of Alma-Ata

The International Conference on Primary Health Care, meeting in Alma-Ata this twelfth day of September in the year Nineteen hundred and seventy-eight, expressing the need for urgent action by all governments, all health and development workers, and the world community to protect and promote the health of all the people of the world, hereby makes the following Declaration:

### I

The Conference strongly reaffirms that health, which is a state of complete physical, mental and social wellbeing, and not merely the absence of disease or infirmity, is a fundamental human right and that the attainment of the highest possible level of health is a most important world-wide social goal whose realization requires the action of many other social and economic sectors in addition to the health sector.

### II

The existing gross inequality in the health status of the people particularly between developed and developing countries as well as within countries is politically, socially and economically unacceptable and is, therefore, of common concern to all countries.

### III

Economic and social development, based on a New International Economic Order, is of basic importance to the fullest attainment of health for all and to the reduction of the gap between the health status of the developing en developed countries. The promotion and protection of the health of the people is essential to sustained economic and social development and contributes to a better quality of life and to world peace.

## IV

The people have the right and duty to participate individually and collectively in the planning and implementation of their health care.

## V

Governments have a responsibility for the health of their people which can be fulfilled only by the provision of adequate health and social measures. A main social target of governments, international organizations and the whole world community in the coming decades should be the attainment by all peoples of the world by the year 2000 of a level of health that will permit them to lead a socially and economically productive life. Primary health care is the key to attaining this target as part of development in the spirit of social justice.

## VI

Primary health care is essential health care based on practical, scientifically sound and socially acceptable methods and technology made universally accessible to individuals and families in the community through their full participation and at a cost that the community and country can afford to maintain at every stage of their development in the spirit of self-reliance and self-determination. It forms an integral part both of the country's health system, of which it is the central function and main focus, and of the overall social and economic development of the community. It is the first level of contact of individuals, the family and community with the national health system, bringing health care as close as possible to where people live and work, and constitutes the first element of a continuing health care process.

## VII

Primary health care:

1. reflects and evolves from the economic conditions and socio-cultural and political characteristics of the country and its communities and is based on the application of the relevant results of social, biomedical and health services research and public health experience;
2. addresses the main health problems in the community, providing promotive, preventive, curative and rehabilitative services accordingly;
3. includes at least: education concerning prevailing health problems and the methods of preventing and controlling them; promotion of food supply and proper nutrition; an adequate supply of safe water and basic sanitation; maternal and child health care, including family planning; immunization against the major infectious diseases; prevention and control of locally endemic diseases; appropriate treatment of common diseases and injuries; and provision of essential drugs;
4. involves, in addition to the health sector, all related sectors and aspects of national and community development, in particular agriculture, animal husbandry, food,

industry, education, housing, public works, communications and other sectors; and demands the coordinated efforts of all those sectors;
5. requires and promotes maximum community and individual self-reliance and participation in the planning, organization, operation and control of primary health care, making fullest use of local, national and other available resources; and to this end develops through appropriate education the ability of communities to participate;
6. should be sustained by integrated, functional and mutually-supportive referral systems, leading to the progressive improvement of comprehensive health care for all, and giving priority to those most in need;
7. relies, at local and referral levels, on health workers, including physicians, nurses, midwives, auxiliaries and community workers as applicable, as well as traditional practitioners as needed, suitably trained socially and technically to work as a health team and to respond to the expressed health needs of the community.

## VIII

All governments should formulate national policies, strategies and plans of action to launch and sustain primary health care as part of a comprehensive national health system and in coordination with other sectors. To this end, it will be necessary to exercise political will, to mobilize the country's resources and to use available external resources rationally.

## IX

All countries should cooperate in a spirit of partnership and service to ensure primary health care for all people since the attainment of health by people in any one country directly concerns and benefits every other country. In this context the joint WHO/UNICEF report on primary health care constitutes a solid basis for the further development and operation of primary health care throughout the world.

## X

An acceptable level of health for all the people of the world by the year 2000 can be attained through a fuller and better use of the world's resources, a considerable part of which is now spent on armaments and military conflicts. A genuine policy of independence, peace, détente and disarmament could and should release additional resources that could well be devoted to peaceful aims and in particular to the acceleration of social and economic development of which primary health care, as an essential, should be allotted its proper share.

***

The International Conference on Primary Health Care calls for urgent and effective national and international action to develop and implement primary health care throughout the world and particularly in developing countries in a spirit of technical cooperation and in keeping with a New International Economic Order. It urges governments, WHO and UNICEF, and other international organizations, as well as multilateral and bilateral agencies, non-governmental organizations, funding agencies, all health workers and the whole world community to support national and international commitment to primary health care and to channel increased technical and financial support to it, particularly in developing countries. The Conference calls on all the aforementioned to collaborate in introducing, developing and maintaining primary health care in accordance with the spirit and content of this Declaration.

## Contributors

*Fred Abbatt*'s early professional experience was as a science teacher and educational technologist. Then, following work in medical education, he became heavily involved in training health workers for primary health care in developing countries. His current major concern is to help governments and NGOs integrate training programmes and plans with health system management needs. To this end, he has formed a company, Health Manpower Systems, which is working with international and bilateral agencies in Africa, the Indian subcontinent, and the Far East. He is the author of several books on training and continuing education for health care workers.

*Harry van Balen*, born in 1930 in Belgium, is a medical doctor who obtained a diploma in Tropical Medicine and Hygiene in 1955 and a Master's degree in Public Health in 1969. He worked previously in health care in general hospital settings in Zaire (1955-1958) and in Rwanda (1959-1968). His major activities included supervision of a medical district, training, and organization of MCH. At present, he is (together with P. Mercenier) head of the Public Health Research and Training Unit at the Institute of Tropical Medicine in Antwerp. Further, he is associate professor in Public Health at the Institute of Tropical Medicine, does research and consultancies in health services organization, and is coordinator of the training in health services organization for the International Course in Health Development in Antwerp.

*Ma. Magdalena A. Barcelon* obtained her M.D. from the University of the Philippines in 1977. She worked with the Rural Missionaries Health Team from 1979 to 1988, first with diocesan community based health programmes in Batangas and Negros Oriental, and later with the national team for services and training. In 1989, she became Executive Director of the Council for Health and Development, a national consortium established to provide services to community-based health programmes and to promote Primary Health Care.

*Chris Bentley* is a British doctor who qualified in Medicine at University College Hospital in 1977. His medical career, leading to Membership of the Royal College of Physicians, was spent working in London teaching hospitals. In 1981, he became medical officer for Save the Children Fund in Northwest Somalia, working initially with refugees, and subsequently helping to develop PHC. In 1983, he joined UNICEF, working as Programme Officer for Health and Nutrition in Somalia. He returned to England in 1988, where he took a Master's degree in Community Medicine. Currently, he is working as Senior Registrar in Public Health Medicine in Bloomsbury Health Authority, London.

*Jarl Chabot* was born in 1947 in the Netherlands. After his medical training, he graduated with an MPH from Ross Institute, London, in 1974. Since that time, he has worked for three years in Angola (1975-1978), and five years in Guinea Bissau (1979-1983). Since 1983 he has been employed by the Royal Tropical Institute (KIT) in Amsterdam, the first three years of which he spent working on a Primary Health Care project in Mali. At present, he is stationed in Amsterdam, where he is in charge of backstopping for PHC projects in the French speaking countries of Africa.

*Dr. A. Mustaque R. Chowdhury* is the Head of the Research and Evaluation Division (RED) of the Bangladesh Rural Advancement Committee (BRAC). Educated at the University of Dhaka (statistics), London School of Economics and Political Science (demography) and the London School of Hygiene and Tropical Medicine (health care epidemiology), Dr. Chowdhury has been working with BRAC since 1977. Here he has worked in various capacities and has helped to develop the Research and Evaluation Division, which is now a large and important division with over 80 staff members. In the early 1980s, he was involved in BRAC's oral rehydration therapy (ORT) programme, which has since developed into the largest ORT programme in the world, reaching more than twelve million mothers. He has published extensively on ORT, immunization, vitamin A, family planning and NGO activities.

*Patricia Dueñas* was born in 1958 in Bogotá, Colombia; she received a nursing degree in 1980 from the Red Cross Nursing Faculty of Rosario University. In 1981, she began her experience in primary health care, working as a public health nurse in the Vaupés Health Service for almost three years. From 1984 to 1986, she was under contract to the Convenio Colombo Holandés (health projects) to work with a primary health care team doing research, design, implementation and evaluation of primary health care models in various Colombian Departamentos (Chocó, Uraba, Guaviare and Vaupés). In 1986 she completed the International Course on Health Development at the Royal Tropical Institute (KIT) in Amsterdam, and received a Master's degree in Public Health. Returning to Colombia in 1987, she returned to her previous job at the Convenio for one year. In 1989 she taught at Cundinamarca University and San Rafael Nursing School. At present, she is under contract to the National University, teaching in the Nursing Faculty in the Management and Education Department and doing research, field work and education of registered nurses in the area of community health.

*Lucy Gilson* is a health economist, interested in developing country issues. She has worked in the planning unit of the Swaziland Ministry of Health, where she was involved in a range of planning activities, including a survey of health sector financing and expenditures. Such work inevitably encouraged thought about health financing, and, after joining the London School of Hygiene and Tropical Medicine in 1986, she took this further by exploring the theoretical bases and practical implications of user fees, a key health financing alternative. Since 1989, she has been seconded to the Swiss Tropical Institute Field Laboratory in southern Tanzania. Here she is coordinating a research project to examine the performance (costs, care offered, patient satisfaction) of rural health units. This involves investigation of both how scarce available resources are used in practice, and how district managers can monitor performance.

*Anita Hardon* was trained as a medical biologist, and is currently a member of the Medical Anthropology Taskforce of the University of Amsterdam. She is involved in a number of research projects concerning drug use in developing countries. She has done health research in both urban and rural communities in the Philippines. This research has resulted, among other publications, in the book *Confronting Ill Health: Medicines, Self-care and the Poor in Manila*, which was recently presented and defended as her PhD thesis.

*Jan-Willem Harnmeijer* has worked as a medical doctor in Africa since 1975, in countries including Tanzania, Kenya, Botswana, Sudan and Zambia. His interest in the problem of financing PHC originates from experience in implementing PHC programmes in deteriorating macro-economic conditions. A member of the PHC unit of The Royal Tropical Institute since 1988, he has a MPH and MSC in Health Planning and Financing.

*Sr. Sara Kaithathara* is a medical mission sister from India with a Master's degree in Public Health. She worked ten years as a nurse and midwife in a hospital, and 18 years in rural areas in India. For the last five years, she has been working in the mountains of Peru.

*Eli Nangawe* is a Tanzanian public health doctor, schooled primarily in Tanzania; he obtained his Master's degree in Public Health at the Royal Tropical Institute (KIT) in Amsterdam in 1987. He has worked, mainly in medicine and public health, with the Maasai for about thirteen years. Currently, he serves as Head of the Health Department in the Lutheran Diocese of Arusha, and in PHC consultancies within and outside Tanzania. His areas of interest are community involvement in health development and education for behavioural change.

*Susan Rifkin* has two degrees in Chinese studies, and became interested in health in developing countries through her work in health care in China. She served as a Health Education Officer in Zambia; then, based in Hong Kong, she spent ten years working with indigenous NGOs, helping to found the Asian Community Health Action Network (ACHAN). She returned to England in 1984, where she works both at the London School of Hygiene and Tropical Medicine and the Liverpool School of Tropical Medicine. Her areas of interest are community participation, urban primary health care, and training materials for health care workers. Most recently, she was team leader for an external evaluation of the WHO Essential Drugs Policy.

*Pieter H. Streefland*, PhD, is head of the Primary Health Care Group of the Royal Tropical Institute in Amsterdam, and Professor of Applied Development Sociology at the University of Amsterdam. He has done extensive research on health and development in South Asia, especially in Bangladesh, India and Nepal.

*Gill Walt* is a Senior Lecturer in Health Policy, and Head of the Health Policy Unit, Department of Public Health & Policy, London School of Hygiene and Tropical Medicine. Her research interests revolve around policy issues in primary health care in the third world, focusing on policy processes (as for example the influence of international agencies and non-governmental organisations in the promotion and implementation of PHC), as well as policy content (e.g. the problems of supervising trained traditional midwives).